HOLISTIC HEALING

SECRETS TO BUILD YOUR IMMUNE SYSTEM AND FIND ANSWERS FOR LONG COVID, CHRONIC FATIGUE SYNDROME, INSOMNIA, EPSTEIN-BARR AND LEAKY GUT

MICHAEL ALCOCK

Copyright © Michael Alcock 2024

All rights reserved. No part of this publication may be reproduced, stored in a retrieval system, or transmitted in any form or by any means, electronic, mechanical, photocopying, recording or otherwise, without prior written permission of the author.

Under no circumstances will any blame or legal responsibility be held against the publisher, or author, for any damages, reparation, or monetary loss due to the information contained within this book. Either directly or indirectly. You are responsible for your own choices, actions, and results.

Legal Notice: This book is copyright protected. This book is for personal use. You cannot amend, distribute sell, use, quote or paraphrase any part, or the content within this book, without the consent of the author or publisher, except for brief quotations in critical reviews or articles.

Disclaimer: Please note the information contained within this document is for educational and entertainment purposes only. All effort has been executed to present accurate, up to date, and reliable, complete information. No warranties of any kind are declared or implied. Readers acknowledge that the author is not engaging in the rendering of legal, financial, medical, or professional advice. The content within this book has been derived from various sources. Please consult a licensed professional before attempting any techniques outlined in this book.

By reading this document, the reader agrees that under no circumstances is the author responsible for any losses, direct or indirect, which are incurred as a result of the use of the information contained within this document, including, but not limited to — errors, omissions, or inaccuracies.

Printed on demand in Australia, United States and United Kingdom.

PREFACE

This book isn't a magic pill you take, and boom, you're cured. It's a shining lighthouse in the storm to guide you away from the rocks and depths of the deep. On your first read through you likely won't take everything in. You may even misinterpret some things. That's OK, you're human. We don't always get it right. The goal here is consistent improvement, not perfection. If you can accept that, the rest should come naturally.

Use this book as a set of boundaries to help direct your lifestyle as you are recovering from your long-haul viral infection. Come back to it when you are going through a rough time. You might find an edge somewhere you didn't see before. Don't be afraid to experiment. You may find in the infinite diversity of the people, food combinations, and environmental factors, a new strategy that works for you.

This book is the book I wish I had when I first got sick. I was a student who had limited nutritional knowledge and resources at my disposal. Everyone I turned to for help couldn't do very much. The methods I prescribe are economical, easy to implement, and totally sustainable. I designed it for people who want to recover fast and return to their normal lives as quickly as possible.

Not everyone has had the same experience as me. Some advice throughout this book is more suited to those with moderate symptoms, particularly the sections on exercise. Please use your discretion and apply what you believe is suitable for you.

CONTENTS

Introduction 5

01.
How Persistent Viruses Work 10

02.
What to stop doing 32

03.
Turbocharge your immune system 67

04.
Healing Food Recipes 94

05.
Nutritional Supplements 117

06.
Advice & Recommendations for People with
Mild to Moderate Long-Haul symptoms .. .. .149

07.
Advice & Recommendations for people with
Severe Long-Haul Symptoms .. .. .153

08.
Medical Treatments.. .. .. .157

09.
Prescription Drugs. .. .. .167

10.
How long will it take to get better? 173

A Final Note.. 177

Acknowledgements . .. .180

References 182

INTRODUCTION

Welcome, dear traveler to the most pragmatic strategy for fighting off persistent viral symptoms! So far, the doctors have probably helped diagnose your condition but offered little advice to get better. You may have tried various urban myths for fighting off infection, but the recurrent symptoms remain. The internet seems to have small nuggets of information scattered here and there, some things working, others wasting your time and money. It's all very confusing and frightening. You may feel isolated, left behind, and can't help wondering whether this could be how the rest of your life will look.

I'm here to tell you there is hope. There is a light at the end of the tunnel. I've been through it all and can say you can take your life back.

Myalgic Encephalomyelitis (ME), chronic fatigue syndrome (CFS), and long Covid (LC) are some of the names doctors call the condition. They're classified in the medical community as idiopathic diseases, a condition that arises suddenly for unknown reasons. Typically, they begin after a viral infection.

Before the Covid-19 pandemic, CFS was the most common diagnosis for persistent symptoms like fatigue and brain fog. An Epstein-Barr virus (EBV) infection was, for many, the catalyst of the condition, though other causes such as Lyme disease, severe acute respiratory syndrome (SARS), and respiratory syncytial virus (RSV) have been known to trigger it as well. Since the pandemic, a new cause of the disease has emerged, with many people who caught Covid continuing to struggle with symptoms and refer to themselves as "long haulers."

Most people recover relatively fast, usually within 1-2 weeks. However, as you no doubt have found, there are those who go on to develop chronic symptoms after the acute phase of a viral infection. Everyone is affected differently, and there isn't a definitive period in which the symptoms will subside.

Depending on the severity of the virus and its strains, surveys estimate between 5-15% of infected people experience symptoms past the acute phase. A quick Google search of the total worldwide infections shows the potentially staggering numbers of people with long-haul symptoms based on those percentages. It's becoming widely accepted that this is a real problem, and Governments are starting to allocate funding to address this, though little progress has been made to understand what's causing the condition.

The severity of the long-haul symptoms ranges significantly. With some people experiencing mild fatigue and brain fog for months, while others become bedridden and incapable of living a normal life.

It's clear to me, even though the pandemic is "over", this condition will continue to be a problem. The virus isn't going away, and new strains are causing outbreaks every few months. Leading to more and more people being at risk of developing life-altering symptoms.

So, how did I get so involved with all of this? When I was 26, I went back to school to get a degree. I was working part-time, living at home, and studying. As I was starting to get into my late twenties, I figured these would probably be the last years I could dedicate a good amount of time to experimenting with my social skills and pushing my physical limits. With the extra time on my hands, I was out socializing as much as I could, riding motorbikes, and making good progress with my strength and fitness. I had always been a reasonably healthy and capable person, but during this time, I really took the opportunity to take things to the next level.

That's when it all came crashing down. A few months after some heavy partying and fitness training, I woke up one morning with the sorest throat I'd ever had. I could barely get myself out of bed, I had a fever so hot it was making me delirious. I'd been sick plenty of times before, but nothing like this. I reached over to my phone and pathetically tried calling my mother, who was in the same house, upstairs, asleep. After seven missed calls, I gave up and lay in agony, trying to soothe myself back to sleep. A few hours later, she woke up and came downstairs to find me in quite the state.

After talking about my symptoms, we decided I needed to see the doctor. He did his usual checks and advised doing a blood test and taking antibiotics in case it was a bacterial infection. Several days later, the doctor called and told me I had glandular fever caused by the Epstein-Barr virus. Being the young, healthy man I was, I was a little dismayed but not overly concerned.

Doing my research on glandular fever, it appeared a 3-month recovery time was standard. I couldn't do very much besides sit on the couch and watch TV, so I took the time to rest as much as I could. I missed out on a few social events here and there, but for a few months, I wasn't too bothered.

Within a month, nearly all my strength and muscular gains had disappeared. Noticeably deflating my ego and self-esteem. Working out had always been a sort of anchor in my life, keeping me grounded and focused. Previously, I was able to take on four subjects at university, work a part-time job, exercise regularly, and have a modest social life. Just about everything from the life I had built was now out of the question, and all I could do was the bare minimum at university, streaming lectures from home for a couple of hours a day.

As I passed the 3-month mark, I had seen mild improvements but wasn't anywhere close to full health. This was when it started to get mentally challenging. "How much longer will it take?" I thought, "I can't keep putting my life on hold; I've got so many things I need to do!" My once burgeoning social life was watching from far away, waving at me to come back. I made some attempts at going out with my friends, but each time I tried, I was exhausted and sometimes couldn't put a sentence together.

My friends and family were supportive at first, but over time, they couldn't understand why I wasn't getting better. I would meet up with friends and go through the same story of feeling tired all the time and coming up with excuses for why I wasn't fun to be around anymore. As months turned into years, I began closing myself off from the world, feeling like something was inherently wrong with me.

It wasn't until I got to the tail end of my degree and saw that the bubble of university life would soon disappear. I realised I needed to take back control of my health or be faced with a life of unemployment and dependency.

I dedicated nearly all my spare time to learning as much as I could about the virus, the immune system, and nutrition to boost my health as much as I could. I spent countless hours researching journal articles, absorbing medical videos on YouTube, and reading books on mystery illnesses. It didn't happen overnight, and I had to make many changes along the way, but with enough grit and optimism, I got my old life back.

For a time, I was enjoying my newfound energy and health again. I could play sports, ride motorbikes, and work out just like I used to, albeit with a few extra years tacked on. But life always has a way of finding new ways to test you. One year later, the Covid-19 disease emerged and blew out into a global pandemic. I managed to evade infection for two years, but after a social basketball game, I became ill and tested positive. My acute infection phase was fairly run of the mill, about two weeks of being bed ridden. However, I soon learned that, like glandular fever, I would be facing another long-haul recovery.

Much like my first round with chronic symptoms, I had to try out new approaches to nutrition and exercise. I was hit with brain fog for about a month and a severe reduction in my physical capacity for three months. My lungs had been damaged from the infection, and any kind of aerobic exercise longer than five minutes would give me a flare-up.

By applying the same principles I learned from glandular fever, I began studying journal articles and reading everything I could online about the virus. I had to tweak a few things in my diet and start all over again with exercise, but once again, I put the puzzle back together. Clawing my way back to health.

After doing research on the condition and learning about what others have been or are still going through, I consider myself one of the lucky ones. I only experienced moderate symptoms, and not everyone has a support network like I had when I was figuring all this out. There are those who have been struggling with severe, persistent symptoms for decades after a viral infection, their lives seemingly changed forever.

I wrote this book to help anyone else who's been afflicted with the condition and can't find anything that works. It can be a horrific position to be in, and I wouldn't wish it upon my worst enemy.

This book is a collection of everything that worked for me and those who've experienced severe symptoms. It's the result of nearly a decade of research, trial, and error, and holding out for hope that one day I could get my life back. My long-haul recovery took years to figure out, and my progress was not consistent. If I had this guide back in 2015, maybe my life would've been different. Fortunately, you've made the right decision to learn more about your health, which will allow you to piece together your own recovery puzzle and avoid many of the pitfalls I made along the way.

CHAPTER 1

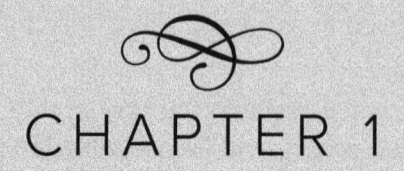

HOW PERSISTENT VIRUSES WORK

This chapter will discuss what causes the disease to occur and how it progresses. If you simply want to learn how to get better, skip ahead. But I would encourage you to read on. Understanding the condition will assist you in your recovery.

All viruses exist for the sole purpose of finding their way into cells which fit with them, converting the cell into a copy of itself, repeating the process exponentially, and spreading to a new host. They aren't alive per se, just a carbon shell with some DNA inside. It's important to understand a virus cannot be "killed"; they stay in the body forever, but they can be deactivated by the immune system.

The time it takes for the immune system to realise what's going on and start fighting back is known as the incubation period. For EBV, it can be one month before symptoms begin to appear; for Covid-19 it appears to vary with each strain. Originally, it was about two weeks, then with new strains, it started coming down to less than one week. The incubation period for Covid appears to be getting shorter, though this could change with new strains down the track.

The length of the immune response period, the time where you "feel" sick, will come down to the individual. Some people are lucky and don't present any symptoms. Others can be completely floored by a virus for weeks but eventually recover. Then there are those who go onto developing chronic symptoms. Many health authorities are now claiming if you're experiencing symptoms past the 3-month mark, you have entered the "long haul" phase.

The health of your immune system, your genetics, and environmental factors determine how your body responds to the infection. There appears to be levels of intensity to the infection based on these factors. The uncertain part, however, is determining a person's risk of developing long-haul symptoms. It seems these factors all play a role in how the virus interacts with the immune system, with some people recovering quickly and others going on to experience chronic symptoms. The levels of chronic symptoms range from being completely bed-ridden to only mildly affected; see below:

Level 1 – Mild symptoms, minor brain fog, and fatigue, can't do high intensity sport, stress tolerance lower.

Level 2 – Moderate symptoms, stronger brain fog and fatigue, reduced hours at work, only light exercise

Level 3 – Severe symptoms, bedridden, 1 hour of activity per day

Level 4 – Very Severe symptoms, loss of muscle function, can't digest food, paralysis.

There has also been research that indicates a previous infection of EBV will increase your chances of developing Long Covid. The new viral infection from Covid distracts the immune system, and EBV reactivates. Placing an enormous burden on your immune response.

While many determined people have tried to figure out what causes chronic symptoms after an acute viral infection, a definitive conclusion has not been agreed upon. There are, however, a few prominent theories that have been studied:

1. **The virus hides in the body, and the immune system can't detect it**

This theory suggests that a virus enters parts of the body where the immune system cannot find it, waiting to be reactivated in the right conditions. I watched a lecture by a doctor talking about EBV and how it enters the bone marrow and hides there until certain conditions are met for it to spring out again. An immune event, such as contracting Covid-19, can reactivate an EBV infection, leading to an overload on a person's immune system from the two active viruses.

This may not be the case for everyone, but one study found a large number of people who were experiencing Long Covid had elevated EBV antibodies in their blood. Meaning their body was fighting off both an EBV and Covid infection at the same time.

It's not certain if this is always the cause of Long Covid, as there have been studies that have found active Covid virus in the gut of people who have persistent symptoms well past their initial infection. EBV can certainly cause long-haul symptoms, and Covid can clearly do the same. What is certain, however, is that both EBV and Covid can evade the immune system for years after the acute infection and continue to cause problems.

2. **The virus changes the body in a way that causes inflammation to persist and other problems to emerge**

A leading theory posits that the high inflammation caused by the virus alters how vital organs function together. The damage caused by the inflammation initiates a cascade of negative feedback loops between normal bodily functions that can spiral downwards if not treated promptly. Some of the disruptions can include the following:

- Vagus Nerve dysfunction
- Mitochondrial dysfunction
- Gut lining dysfunction leading to gut dysbiosis.
- Thyroid dysfunction
- Brain dysfunction
- Immune system dysfunction
- Oxygen transport dysfunction

Each of these dysfunctions have a connection with each other. As the high inflammation spreads everywhere, the entire body is at risk of viral-induced damage, leading to one function breaking down, and another and another, and so on. The human body is a series of interconnected systems operating together. If one begins to deteriorate, there are flow on effects to all organs.

The weakened state of the body prompts the viral infection to run rampant. The normal mechanisms of lowering inflammation become impaired, which in turn leads to further organ damage. The highly inflamed state leads to acidosis of the blood, causing hypoxia (low oxygen) and high levels of lactate in the muscles. Meanwhile, the production of the energy-carrying molecules found in cells, Adenosine Triphosphate (ATP), goes down due to an increase in histamine and reactive oxygen species (ROS) that damage the mitochondria.

Many people have reported their nervous system being affected; severe cases report developing Dysautonomia and its variant Postural Orthostatic Tachycardia Syndrome (POTS). This is where automatically controlled functions such as heart rate, blood pressure, and digestion are compromised. Common symptoms of this condition are dizziness, fainting, and brain fog from the mildest of activities.

Another common dysfunction is Mast Cell Activation Syndrome. Where some of the body's immune cells (the mast cells) become hyperactive and release histamine causing hives, itching, abdominal pain, and brain fog.

In severe cases, the high inflammation damages the endothelial layer of the blood vessels, which is responsible for maintaining the health and functionality of the cardiovascular system. If sustained, the body forms micro clots to patch up the damaged blood vessels and can induce arterial plaquing. The dysfunctional blood vessels become unable to deliver oxygen and essential nutrients to the tissues, accelerating the severe downward spiral of fatigue.

Perhaps the most sinister of the dysfunctions is the damage done to the intestinal lining. The highly inflamed gut lining can result in gut dysbiosis, causing nutrient absorption to become impaired. Easy to digest foods cause bloating or simply are not absorbed by the body at all. This creates nutrient deficiencies with even with a moderately healthy diet.

Another issue is short-chain fatty acids and various bacteria, which aren't supposed to leave the gut, seep through the damaged gut lining, and enter the blood stream. These make their way up to the brain and increase neuroinflammation (brain fog).

3. **The virus damages vital organs such as, but not limited to, the Brain, Liver, and Heart**

This is perhaps the most devastating theory put forward. There is tangible medical evidence that Covid-19 causes scarring in the lungs, which I can personally attest to. I've also heard of people losing hearing in one ear and having their sense of taste and smell vanish or be altered horribly.

Then there are the blood clots that the high inflammation causes. These are essentially body wide amyloid-fibrin-calcium deposits to build up in the blood vessels, preventing your blood from delivering nutrients, oxygen, and fatty acids to the tissues. In turn, causing more damage to vital organs. This is usually where a person's body becomes so far gone that normal methods of recovery fail to work, and the downward spiral of fatigue accelerates.

As someone who has lived through the experience for many years with two particularly nasty viruses, my best take is that all three of these theories are applicable. The acute immune response clears away most of the easy to find pathogens (an infectious agent causing disease), but any impairment to this response allows portions of the virus to remain. Causing persistent inflammation, immune dysfunctions, and eventually, damage to vital organs and the vascular system. Viruses have also been known to mutate inside the body, requiring your immune system to "retrain" its detectors to find the new strains of the virus.

As the condition is complicated, and was relatively unstudied until Covid-19, professional awareness and training for this condition isn't commonplace. Because of this knowledge gap, misdiagnosis or under diagnosis can occur, leaving people at best getting better very slowly, or at worst spiraling towards total dependency.

Explaining how a virus hides from the immune system is very complicated and not completely understood. I've combined my personal experience with medical research to have a general understanding of it. I've summarised what I like to call the "Pest" analogy below.

The "Pest" Analogy

Think of the immune response being like a household pest eradication. One day, you find a nest of nasty critters inside your house, and you decide to book a pest extermination expert to clear out the problem. The expert arrives at your house and begins working. He assesses the situation and decides to use a poison that, in the past, has worked quite well. He goes ahead and sprays every nasty critter he sees, leaves some poison bait to eliminate any offspring and calls it a day. As it happens, only 40% of the pests died from the initial response, so the pest expert must be called back to reassess the situation, purchase new poison, and complete the process once again.

How effective the expert will be at his job depends on a few things. Has the owner of the house made it easy for the pests to propagate? Has the house been regularly cleaned with quality products and all maintenance taken care of? How many pest prevention measures were taken when building the house? Are there any ongoing issues that might make it easy for pests to breed?

Now, you're probably thinking if a pest control expert needed to keep coming back to eliminate the infestation, he wouldn't have a very successful business. Word would get around that they weren't effective, and the market would punish them. Unfortunately, as humans, we don't have that luxury. Our only pest control expert available is the immune system. We can, however, work with our immune system to support and strengthen it.

The bad feelings you get from the immune response can be compared to a battlefield inside your body. It's kind of like when soldiers are storming into a village occupied by an invader. The ensuing conflict prevents any of the normal day-to-day activities from working very well. It's important to let the soldiers deal with the invaders as best they can, or the battle could drag on and expose more civilians to crossfire. Think of eating healthy foods as giving your soldiers the best supplies to fight the invaders. Medications and supplements are like upgrading the weapons of your soldiers. Allowing yourself to rest is like vacating the village to let them fight without getting in the way. It's a good sign when you feel sick and tired. It means your immune system is doing its job, and you are progressing with your recovery. It can be incredibly inconvenient to your life; believe me, I know. But it's so important you surrender to your body and let it do its job.

Modern science has not devised a method of testing the level of persistent viral infection inside someone. There are tests available to detect whether an antibody to a virus is present, and more advanced tests to determine the level of antibodies in your blood. A test that measures where and how bad an infection is has not been developed, to my knowledge, at least.

As discussed earlier, people with severe cases experience significant damage all over their body to the point where supporting the immune system with rest and healthy eating is not always sufficient to prompt recovery. The body has gotten to a point where nutrient absorption and vasculature damage is so bad that external intervention is required.

Why do some people only get mildly sick, and others become bedridden?

There are a number of reasons why some people only get a few sniffles while others barely have enough energy to get out of bed. Besides the factors in a person's control, such as the quality of food, the level of stress, and the health of their immune system, the other factors are a person's age, being the older someone is, the weaker their immune system tends to get, and whether they have any pre-existing health problems. For example, diabetes, or any other immunocompromising diseases.

Then there are the genetic predispositions a person may be born with for high inflammation and being more susceptible for a weakened immune response, which nobody has any control over.

Have you ever noticed how some people are more highly strung than others? I, for one, have always been a fidgeter and can be prone to burn out faster than the average person. This is because of certain genes I have that determine my baseline adrenaline levels. Because my level of adrenaline is higher from the get-go, I am more likely to go hard at the beginning of a task but have less endurance overall. This places me and anyone else with this genotype at a higher risk of being run down and susceptible to infection.

Another set of genes that contribute to a higher risk are the inflammatory response mechanisms. Histamine, an inflammatory molecule, is released from a variety of sources within the body, such as interleukin cytokines IL-1B and TNF-a. Everyone has these genes, but some people have gene variants that promote a stronger histamine response than others. Placing them at a higher risk of chronic inflammation.

You may have heard of Covid causing a "cytokine storm", where the immune response to the virus is so overwhelming that the body dumps cytokines everywhere to stave off the infection. Unfortunately, this highly inflammatory state leads to other issues, and isn't always effective at neutralizing a viral infection.

Out of curiosity, I purchased a DNA test a few years ago to get a better understanding of what I was made up of. It showed my baseline adrenaline levels are naturally high, and I'm at a moderately higher risk of developing chronic inflammation. This helps to explain why I kept getting injured during sport when I was growing up and why I had a hard time recovering from EBV and Covid.

Common Misconceptions about CFS and Long Covid

1. "It's all in your head"

A horrible accusation that can get even the most patient person infuriated. Gaslighting leaves someone feeling powerless and isolated. It's a complete fabrication; it diminishes the chance of their recovery and putting them at risk for social withdrawal.

When I went back to my doctor, years after I was first infected, I was told that I was experiencing a type of phantom pain caused by the virus. Which, in his mind, was no longer causing any real issues. He prescribed an antidepressant that focused on neuropathic pain. Taking the drug, I did feel less anxiety, but it made me dopey and sedated. I couldn't stay focused on anything or perform at my job. What's the point of taking a drug if it destroys your zest for life?

2. "There's nothing physically wrong with you"

While doctors may be doing their best with conventional methods of testing, accurately diagnosing the condition requires a far more in-depth approach. The sad reality is that this becomes a form of unintentional gaslighting, as the patient feels isolated and left behind.

I remember watching a documentary on people suffering from long Covid. There was a panel of doctors speaking about the tests they had performed on a young man who had debilitating fatigue and brain fog. One doctor sincerely proclaimed he couldn't find anything wrong with him. The look on the young man's face said it all.

In the specialist fields, information about the condition is slowly beginning to disseminate. However, in most cases, the average GP has not received any education about testing or treatment. If your regular doctor isn't being helpful, I find it is better to smile and move on then pushing for further assistance. It simply isn't worth the energy to persuade them something is wrong.

3. "Have you tried exercising?"

You think I haven't?!? I believe most people understand the importance of exercise and how it can improve your health. For a healthy person, exercise is great. For a person with long Covid/CFS, even the slightest over-exertion can knock you back to bed for days.

The problem is this condition is it's unlike any normal illness. The inflammation feedback loop in your cells has changed how your body responds to exercise. You may not feel it straight away, but the risk of crashing for days is very high.

Before I was sick, I was incredibly fit. Going for 50km bike rides every weekend and doing calisthenics throughout the week. Even after months of rest, I struggled to return to light activities.

Sometimes, when I was feeling a little better, I took it as a sign that I could start pushing myself like I used to. More often than not, I would experience a devastating bout of PEM.

As we'll discuss later, the body needs to be taken care of properly before returning to exercise. The conventional advice of waiting a week or two after illness to return to exercise is dangerous for people who are at risk of developing the condition.

4. "You have to want to get better!"

Trust me. Everyone with this condition wants nothing more than to get better. I will admit that there is a mental aspect to recovering; you need to stay positive. There was nothing I wanted more while I was sick than to get better and feel normal again.

Those who caught EBV or Covid and were fine shortly afterwards don't understand why we're effected like this. For their whole lives, being sick has been a minor inconvenience that lasts two weeks at the most. It is frustrating to hear comments like this. It's tempting to snap and blast them with a verbal attack, but this won't serve any purpose.

Perhaps one positive that comes from this is that the condition puts life in perspective. Those who had extensive social lives are quickly shown who their real friends are. Millionaires who once lived the high life are humbled by no longer having the energy to enjoy the activities they once did. If you don't have your health, you really don't have much at all.

The Adrenal Glands

I don't want to give you a complete lesson in human biology, mainly because it would be an overload of information, and you'd get bored quickly. However, it is important to understand how certain parts of your body work in order to mentally accept what's going on. The Adrenal Glands are a miracle of nature. Acting like the pharmacy for the body, producing all the anti-inflammatory and steroid hormones we need to keep ourselves alive and fed. They sit on top of the kidneys, as can be seen in the picture below.

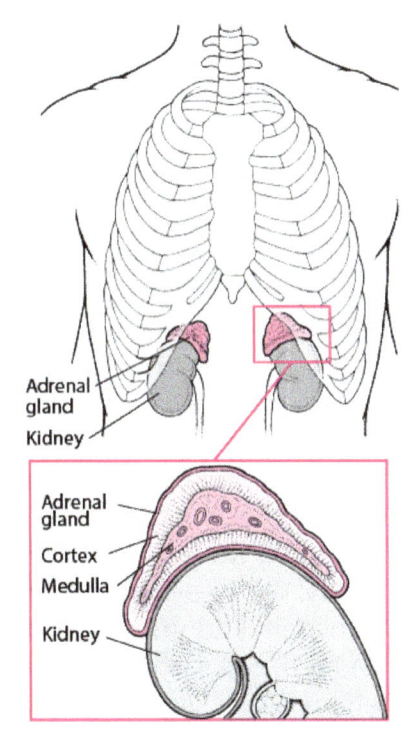

It's important to understand any Pharmacy can run out of stock if not managed correctly. High levels of repeated stress and poor nutrition will overwork these glands, putting the body into a state known as "adrenal fatigue". Have you ever gone through a highly stressful period and just wanted to do nothing for several days afterward? This is a sign of mild adrenal fatigue, and it can get worse the longer the stress isn't alleviated.

Your level of recovery will determine how much stress and activity you can tolerate. When the body is infected with a virus or bacteria, the level of stress increases, demanding more nutritional resources to fight off the infection. This process causes inflammation, brain fog, and fatigue. In this state, it is unlikely you'll have much capacity to deal with everyday life. If there is a life-threatening situation, the body would do its best to divert any available energy to producing adrenaline. This will tax the adrenals significantly, and a long period of fatigue will follow afterward.

It's crucial after periods of stress that the adrenals are supported by resting and eating healthy food. If there is no nutritional support, or it's not possible to rest, the body will remain in "stress mode" as the irritation from fighting off the virus keeps stress high. This presents as the symptom of insomnia, where even though you may be harrowingly tired, sleep never comes because the adrenals have not been supported properly and cannot turn off. It's one of life's paradoxes, whereby being so tired and needing sleep, the most important thing your body needs, is not permitted.

One of the difficulties of modern-day life is, even with its conveniences, our level of baseline stress has never been higher. Adrenal fatigue is common for people even without a persistent viral infection. Our fast-paced lives are bombarded by the highs and lows of social media. You turn on the news, and it's a competition to see what the worst thing is that's happened in the world today. We've eliminated the life-threatening stressors from wild animals and improved our technology to keep us sheltered and fed. But in their place, we've increased mental stress. Sometimes, watching your favourite comfort TV show or reading a book are just what we need to unplug and let our minds settle down.

While adrenal fatigue is serious, it is more of a problem in people with only mild to moderate long-haul symptoms. People who can still participate in daily life though are no longer capable of intense activity or exercise. Typically, because they can still go to work and attend to their duties while fighting off a persistent virus, they put themselves at risk for burning out.

For people with severe long-haul symptoms, the pervasive damage done to your body will be causing extreme fatigue. Supporting the adrenal glands is important but will not yield the same results as those with mild to moderate symptoms.

The Lymphatic System

You've probably heard of the cardiovascular and nervous system of the human body. The Lymphatic system is like these in that it covers most of your body, but its function differs significantly. The lymphatic system is like the "sewer" of the body, where waste material from the immune system and blood is processed and expelled.

It works by circulating fluid called lymph that carries white blood cells and waste products throughout the body by way of lymphatic vessels. The lymph is filtered by lymph nodes, which contain immune cells that help to identify and neutralise pathogens such as bacteria and viruses.

After the filtering process, the lymph is returned to the bloodstream through the thoracic duct, a large vessel that connects to the veins near the heart.

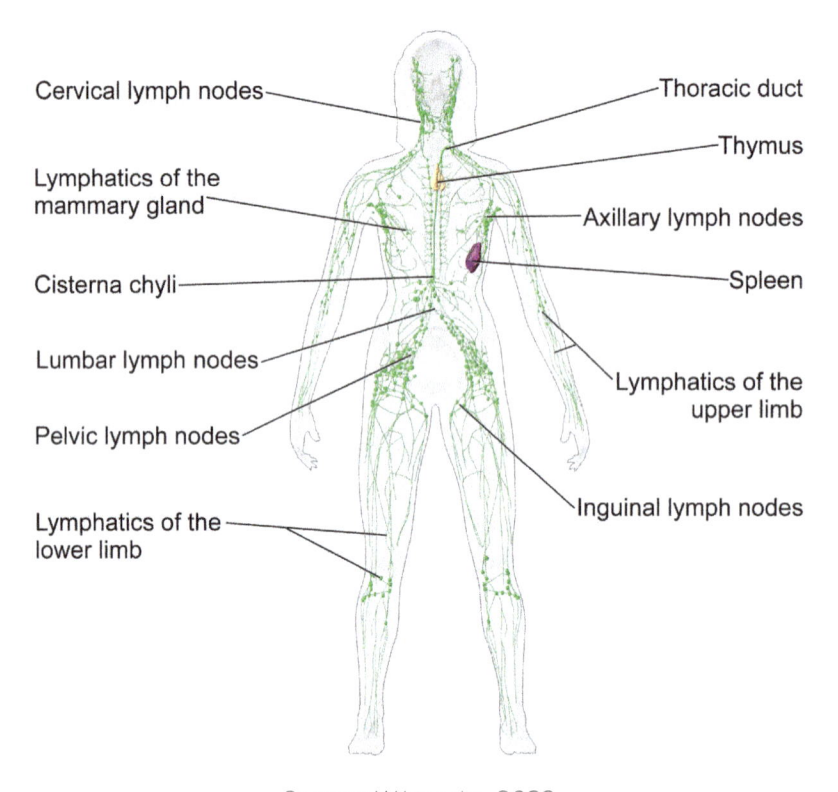

Cervical lymph nodes
Thoracic duct
Thymus
Lymphatics of the mammary gland
Axillary lymph nodes
Cisterna chyli
Spleen
Lumbar lymph nodes
Lymphatics of the upper limb
Pelvic lymph nodes
Inguinal lymph nodes
Lymphatics of the lower limb

Source: Wikipedia. 2023.

Unlike the cardiovascular system, which has the heart to pump everything around, the lymphatic system has no means of automatic circulation. It must be done manually. To drain the lymphatic vessels and glands of lymph build-up, there are several methods you can enact:

1. Exercise: Physical activity helps to stimulate lymph flow by contracting muscles and increasing circulation. It doesn't have to be much; simple activities such as walking, stretching, or Yoga can help get lymph moving.

2. Massage: Gentle massage or lymphatic drainage therapy can increase the flow of lymph around the body and lower your stress levels. This may be necessary for those with severe symptoms and cannot leave their bed.

3. Hydration: Drinking plenty of water keeps your lymph vessels as hydrated as possible to keep things moving.

4. Deep Breathing: Taking deep, diaphragmatic breaths can stimulate lymph flow by increasing pressure in the abdominal area.
5. Avoid tight clothing: Tight clothing can restrict lymph flow and lead to fluid retention.

Eating clean, nutritious food will strengthen the immune response in your lymphatic system, preventing swelling in lymph glands and reducing blockages when a pathogen enters the body.

EBV just so happens to target the lymphatic system, part of the reason why it takes so long to recover from the virus. It's one thing to have a virus inhabit your sinuses but to have it disrupt one of the immune system's most important tools makes it a very serious infection to deal with.

There were times while I was recovering where I couldn't do basic exercise for a week. While I might've needed the time off, I did start to feel a little clogged up. Going for a gentle bike ride in the sun, phlegm would start to drain down from my sinuses. This is a sign of the waste fluid being excreted from my body. Ever had a runny nose? It's caused by mucus build up from an infection, but if it's a clear fluid that's coming out, it's a sign your lymphatic system is draining out.

While EBV targets this system, Covid tends to go for the respiratory system initially, causing all sorts of breathing and lung capacity issues. Any kind of limitation on your oxygen intake will severely limit how much exercise you can do. Exercise is generally the most accessible way of circulating lymph, but while your lungs are recovering, use other less demanding ways of pumping out this system from some of the examples earlier.

When any kind of exercise isn't feasible, massage is the best way to circulate lymph throughout your body. Generally, a lighter massage touch is preferred for lymphatic drainage.

The "Ceiling" Principle

An important notion for those with mild to moderate symptoms is to understand the recovery "ceiling" principle. When you're infected with any kind of pathogen, your body will react by ramping up your immune system activity and use most of its energy in identifying and neutralising the invaders. In this acute phase of the response, your general capacity for any kind of activity is greatly reduced. The "ceiling" on how much you can do is quite low. The recovery ceiling is characterised by the limit of how much stress and exercise you can tolerate. As you recover, the ceiling begins to rise, and your limits improve. At any time you try to exceed the ceiling of your limits, you put yourself at risk of crashing, also known as post-exertional malaise (PEM). This is your body's way of saying you broke the rules; now you must pay the price.

In a perfect world, where your immune system is strong, you have little stress in your life, and you're getting all the nutrition you need to support your recovery, the rate at which you recover would look something in the graph below:

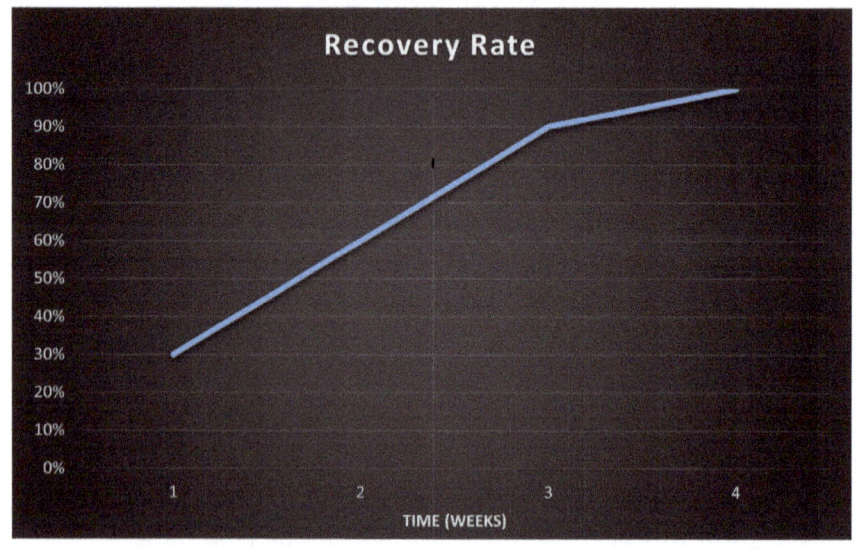

Recovery Rate

The first two weeks knock you around a little bit. You're bed ridden for a week or two, you don't want to leave the house, but the recovery is consistent, and by about week three, you start feeling like you could get back out there.

Now let's look at someone who might've been quite stressed out when they got infected, maybe had a few roadblocks to their recovery, and had to return to their daily activities shortly after the acute infection phase.

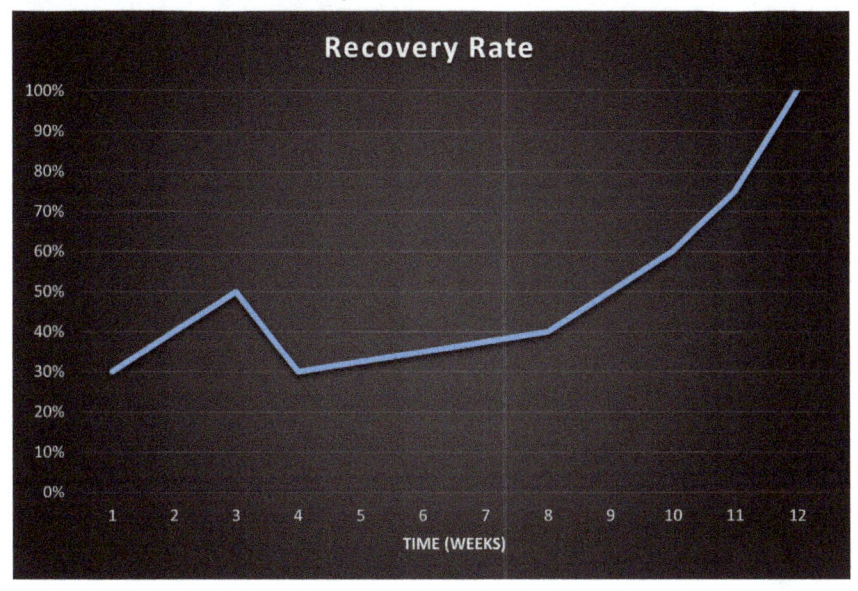

Recovery Rate

You can see the speed of recovery is much slower to begin with, and the sudden drop in recovery is caused by a stressful period at work. These kinds of events don't always just slow the recovery down; you actively go backwards in your progress because the virus has had a chance to reassert itself.

Now let's look at someone who has a lifestyle with multiple roadblocks and regularly goes through high-stress periods but keeps a reasonably healthy diet.

Recovery Rate

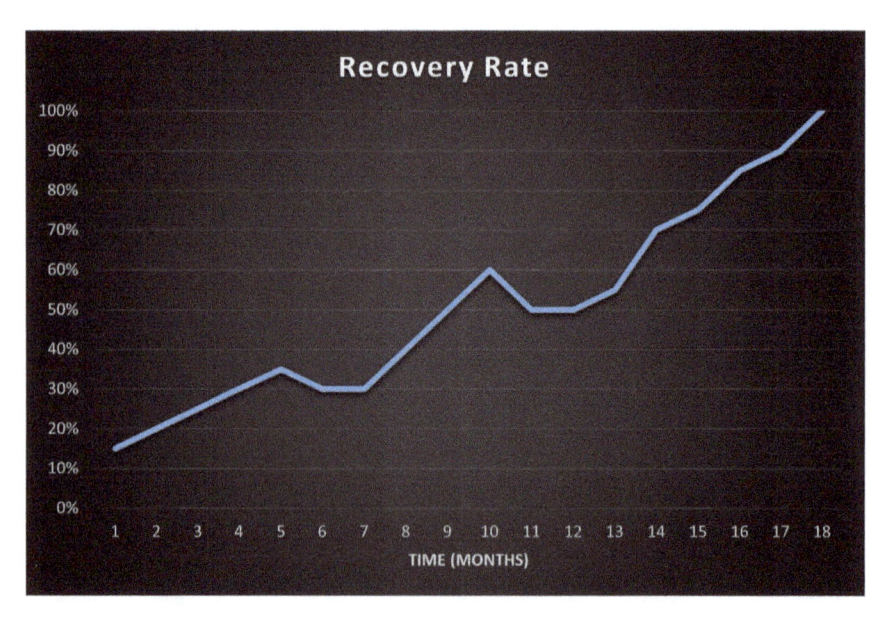

(Chart: Recovery Rate percentage over Time in Months, showing an overall upward trend from ~15% at month 1 to ~100% at month 18, with setbacks around months 5-7 and 10-11.)

You'll notice the time is in **months**, not weeks. This kind of person likely received a high viral load from the onset of infection, leaving their immune system with a massive job. They do their best to eat well but are consistently going through setbacks. This is a classic case of "long-haul" symptoms, but at the very least, they are getting better.

Many people are unknowingly putting up roadblocks to their recovery and failing to provide their immune system with the resources it needs to wage war on the virus. They feel like they're improving at a snail's pace, taking months to show any progress, and even going through periods of regression.

These three examples don't cover everyone's situation. There are people who feel like they've been getting worse for months, and the slightest push can send them to bed for days at a time.

Persistent viruses are always waiting for the right moment to strike, such as when your immune system is weakened or when you consume foods that trigger inflammation and histamine. A commonly sinister trait of many of these persistent viruses is also to turn off the uptake of important vitamin receptors in the body, such as Vitamin D. Further diminishing your immune systems resources and adding to the inflammation storm.

It's important to note that there is not **one single thing** you need to stop or start doing to recover. It's a series of 1% efforts that have a cumulative effect on your health. This is not the news I'm sure you were hoping to hear. The advertising world has conditioned us to expect a magic pill that will heal us from any kind of ailment. This is incredibly convenient; however, in reality, this kind of thinking will not get you very far.

I've felt the pain, grief, and anger from being sick for a long time. There's a lot of frustration that comes from nothing seeming to work, and anxiety from the uncertainty of what the future will look like. It takes real strength to change your life and get better, but I know for a fact that if you want something hard enough and are terrified of staying the same, nothing will stop you from getting it.

Now that you know some of the fundamentals of the immune system and the nature of the condition, let's start going through some of the fundamentals for improving your health. Before we get into specific detail, I'll go over the framework that will govern how you will approach your recovery. Depending on your level of long-haul symptoms, your rate of response will vary.

Everyone's health situation is inherently different, a vitamin C deficiency may be holding you back, but for someone else it could be mould exposure keeping them unwell. Restoring health is a process of elimination, starting with the basics, and trying new things one by one to see if it is pertinent to you.

Refer to this whenever you are going through a tough time or feel a little stumped as to why you're not making progress.

The Framework for Recovery

1. Remove as many roadblocks as possible to your recovery
   - These are what keep the virus activated in the body, allowing inflammation to occur and disruptions to your normal bodily functions to persist.
2. Give your body the resources it needs to support recovery
   - Your diet should consist of natural, whole foods and not rely on supplements
   - Depending on the level of your symptoms, you may need to consult with a licensed physician on some of the treatments detailed in the "Advice for people with Severe Long-Haul Symptoms" chapter to give your immune system a good boost for recovery
   - Get a DNA test to determine food allergies, genotypes, and inflammation markers
   - If you believe you have gut issues, then a stool test will help identify what's going on inside your gut
   - The body needs nutrients to keep the immune system functioning properly. It also needs resources to repair itself and lower the acidity of your blood caused by the virus
3. Lower Stress in all its forms
   - Any kind of intense stress will turn off the immune system and increase blood acidity levels, allowing the virus to assert itself
4. Give yourself time to recover
   - Depending on how bad your condition is, recovery may take a while. It's important to be patient with your body and keep nourishing it effectively

In the next chapters, I'll talk about the things you need to stop doing that are holding back your recovery and the changes you can make to start turbocharging your immune system.

CHAPTER SUMMARY: HOW PERSISTENT VIRUSES WORK

- Incubation periods can vary from virus to virus.
- There are many theories for persistent symptoms, though it's likely caused by the viral infection triggering a cascade of negative feedback loops in the body.
- Some people have a pre-disposition for high inflammation and stress in the body, leading to higher chances of blood acidosis, which leads to severe endothelial dysfunction
- The Adrenal Glands are a vital component of your immune system and inflammatory response. Take good care of them.
- The Lymphatic System is like the sewer treatment plant of the body, filtering your blood for all sorts of pathogens.
- The Ceiling Principle describes the upper limit of your energy and stress capacity. Breaking through the "ceiling" will cause you to crash.
- The condition is grossly misunderstood in the medical profession. Exercise caution when discussing it with a doctor.

CHAPTER 2

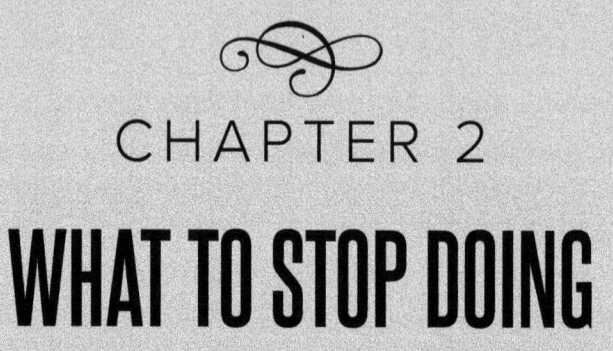

WHAT TO STOP DOING

The items in this chapter have been classified into three tiers of avoidance. Some of the items will have devastating effects on your recovery, whereas others will only have an effect for a day or two. The state of your condition will determine the severity of how each item will impact your health.

As you get better, you may be able to tolerate life's indulgences, such as alcohol, coffee, and sugar, a little more. However, with the objective of recovering as fast as possible, it's ideal that all items be avoided for as long as you can. The common theme with these items is they either deplete the body of nutrients, raise blood acidity & histamines, increase inflammation, or do a combination of all of them.

I would be lying if I said I was a complete saint and abstained from everything on this list while I was recovering. The occasional indulgence or mistake won't be the end of the world, so don't stress too much. By having a greater awareness of the roadblocks to your recovery, you can make better decisions for yourself.

The tiers are described as the following:

Tier 1 - Avoid at all costs whether you're healthy or sick

Tier 2 - Remove from your life completely until you're better

Tier 3 - Not horrible, but should be avoided most of the time

What you'll come to learn are the patterns of how you're feeling and recognising the limits of your current recovering ceiling. For example, if you've had a rough week at work, maybe had a few too many sugary snacks, then going to that party on the weekend and drinking alcohol probably isn't a good idea.

Think of your health like a bank. When you're sick, there's little money inside, and whatever is being deposited will quickly be spent on fighting the virus. Any kind of stress or high-intensity activity will also wipe out any of the money. To build up the bank balance, it takes careful management and frugal spending. Over time, with enough patience, the balance will increase to a point where you can make a few withdrawals from time to time without getting into trouble.

There are several items on this list that should always be avoided. Without it mattering whether you're sick or healthy. In this chapter, we'll explore the roadblocks holding you back from a swift recovery.

Food containing MSG (Tier 1)

Monosodium Glutamate (MSG) is a flavour enhancer used in processed food, take away, and by restaurants. It's commonly found in snack foods, seasonings, processed meats, frozen meals, and salad dressings. In a nutshell, it's a cheap and easy food additive that most people can't tell if it's been used.

Have you ever ordered some yummy takeaway for dinner and had trouble sleeping that night? That's a symptom of an MSG overdose. Besides giving you a bad night's sleep, it can also cause headaches, vomiting, night sweats, and chest pain. If you see any of the names below on an ingredient list, you can probably assume MSG has been added.

- Hydrolysed Vegetable Protein
- Autolyzed Yeast
- Glutamic Acid
- Sodium Caseinate
- Textured Protein
- Natural Flavouring
- Spice Extract
- Carrageenan

As you can see, there are many alternative names MSG can be labelled as. For a healthy person, it can take a lot before any symptoms appear. However, for a person recovering from a persistent virus, it's just another thing the liver and lymphatic system must process.

It's one thing to read the ingredient list in a supermarket but another thing to get a straight answer out of a restaurant. Because of its divisive reputation, few restaurants will own up to putting MSG in their food. After all, anybody who is asking about it is likely trying to avoid it! Some of the tell-tale signs are places that have bad reviews, aren't getting much traffic, and the quality of the primary ingredients is poor. MSG is used as a cost saver to maximize the taste of food. In many cases, you won't know for sure you've eaten food with it until later that night when you're having trouble getting to sleep or keep waking up through the night.

Nutritional Gaps in your diet (Tier 1)

I remember before I got sick, I thought eating broccoli, some carrots, and a bit of fruit was all you needed to stay healthy. Boy, what a revelation it was when I began to let go of that attitude.

There certainly are vitamins and minerals that you need to focus on when recovering from a viral infection, but having a deficiency in ANY of the vitamins and minerals will impede the rate at which you recover. Every vitamin and mineral is important and any kind of deficiency will weaken your immune system.

Unfortunately, supplementation will only get you so far. Many vitamin pills and powders use synthetic vitamins and minerals which are poorly absorbed by the human body. The production process also removes enzymes and other significant properties from food, which are highly beneficial to our bodies.

To give you a basic overview, every vitamin and mineral we need serves multiple interconnected roles in the body, ranging from energy production, helping the immune system and relaxing your muscles. A deficiency in any of them will, over a period, cause a drop in energy and vitality. The trick is identifying where you're falling short in your diet early and knowing what to focus on to plug any of the gaps.

The trouble with covering all your nutritional needs is that there are so many parts to worry about. Most people, including myself, have difficulty deciding what food they feel like on any given day, let alone what nutrition they need to keep them healthy. Unless you have your own private chef and nutritionist, you're going to have to learn the basics of the nutritional content of food to keep yourself healthy.

Cronometer is a free tool available online (Google Cronometer) that allows you to list the foods you've eaten in a day and shows how close you are to hitting your nutritional needs. It's a great tool that's easy to use and quickly shows what you're doing well in and where you need to improve. Not only that, but it also tells you the types of foods you need to eat to get specific vitamins and minerals.

In the next chapter, I will talk about this more, but for now, understand that any kind of nutritional gap will have a negative effect on your recovery.

Smoking and Vaping (Tier 1)

Should go without saying these days, but I'll mention it anyway. Any kind of smoking and vaping must be stopped immediately as all these products will most certainly contain harmful chemicals and carcinogens that will damage your lungs and be absorbed into your bloodstream.

Mould (Tier 1)

Mould in the environment is toxic to humans if inhaled. You've probably seen fruit or vegetables left out for too long and seen them turn yellow and green. That's what mould looks like. It's caused by tiny spores floating around from the outside world finding either decaying foods or cold damp areas which have poor ventilation. The spores find their way to these spots and begin to propagate from the conditions, releasing bacteria and particulate matter as it breaks down what it's attached to. It is possible to detect these toxic compounds with your nose, though the smell must be quite strong before you notice it. At that point the mould has likely grown significantly and will already be causing health issues. In most cases, you won't even know you're being exposed, as mould is often hidden away in dark and damp locations. If exposed daily, it's likely you'll be run down and fall ill frequently without changing anything else in your routine.

To give you a brief overview of how it affects people, it starts when we breathe in the toxins and they enter our respiratory system. For some, this causes allergic reactions, but overall, it depletes our immune system and in bad cases, causes neurological problems. If you're an asthmatic, you also have a much high susceptibility to being affected by mould. You can do everything you can to bolster your immune system with supplements and by eating well. But at the end of the day, the mould will come out on top and keep you down. The best option is always to identify where you are being exposed to mould and either remove yourself from that area or eliminate the mould.

I learned this lesson the hard way by buying a grotty used car at a bargain price. It had a bad smell coming from the A/C system, but I thought I was really clever, and I reckoned I could clean it up. I spent hundreds of dollars on cleaning products and slaved away for a dozen weekends trying to flush it all out. Sadly, the mouldy smell always came back. For the six months I owned it, I was sick for nearly a week for every one of those months. My work colleagues thought I was a joke, and I was burning through my sick leave. In the end, I swallowed my pride and sold the car to a wrecker for a substantial loss.

If you live in an area where it rains regularly and gets humid, you can bet that mould will be a problem if not taken care of early. At the time of writing, here in Australia, we'd recently been through a particularly heavy rain season, which brought on an outbreak of mould. Just about every building was hit hard with mould growth. Ceilings, walls, cupboards, outdoor patios, and roof gutters were all covered in green, black mould growth. Real Estate agents for rentals were inundated with professional mould removal requests, and many people were forced to be exposed to the toxic spores.

If you feel comfortable removing mould yourself, there are a few ways to go about it. Always wear gloves and a heavy-duty face mask when using cleaning chemicals to avoid skin and lung irritations. The most common method of removal is to scrub the affected area with vinegar, making sure to wipe off all the growth and thoroughly rinsing off. The vinegar solution should be 1 part vinegar and three parts water. If it gets on your clothes, towels, or bed linen, give it a wash and put it outside into the sunlight to dry for several hours. Sunlight is a great disinfectant.

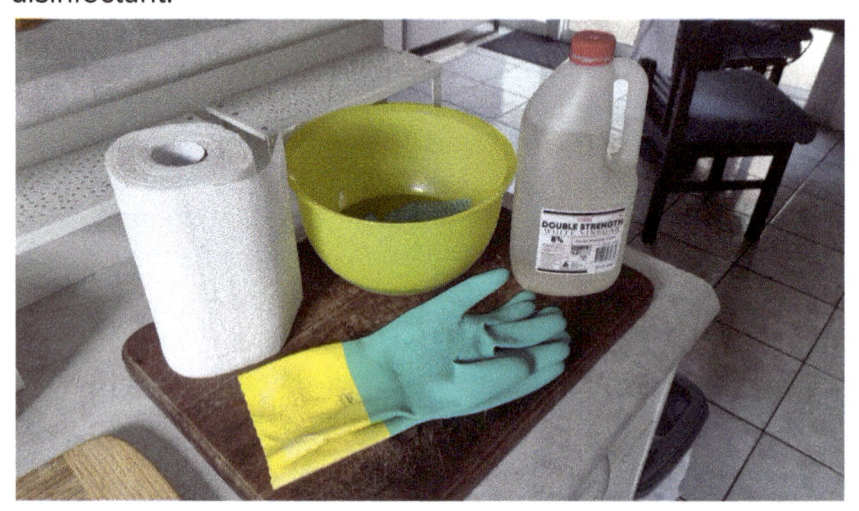

It is possible to get air sprays to get to hard-to-reach areas, but they usually require specialised equipment for dispersal. If you're not confident you can easily take care of it, seek a professional's help. It's just not worth the impact it could have on your health.

You can Google what mould looks like, but here are a few examples:

HOLISTIC HEALING

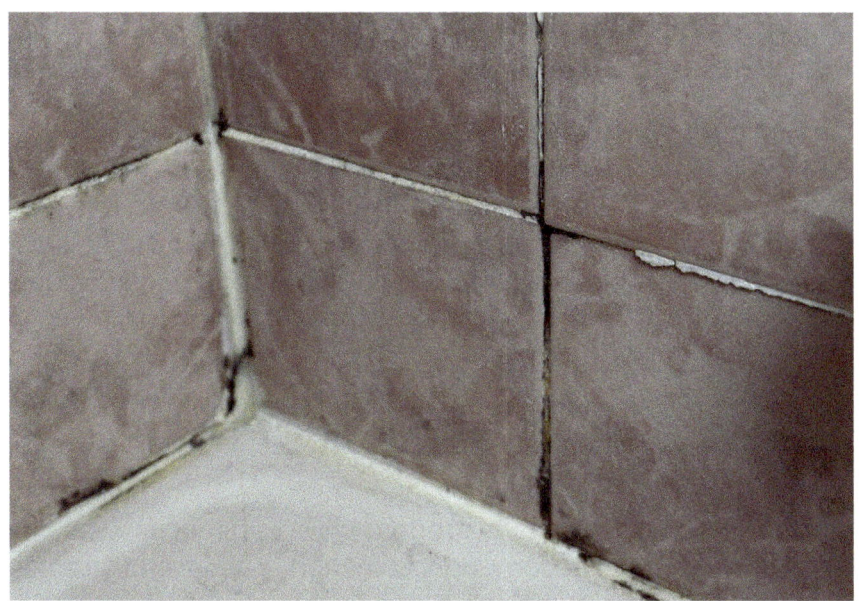

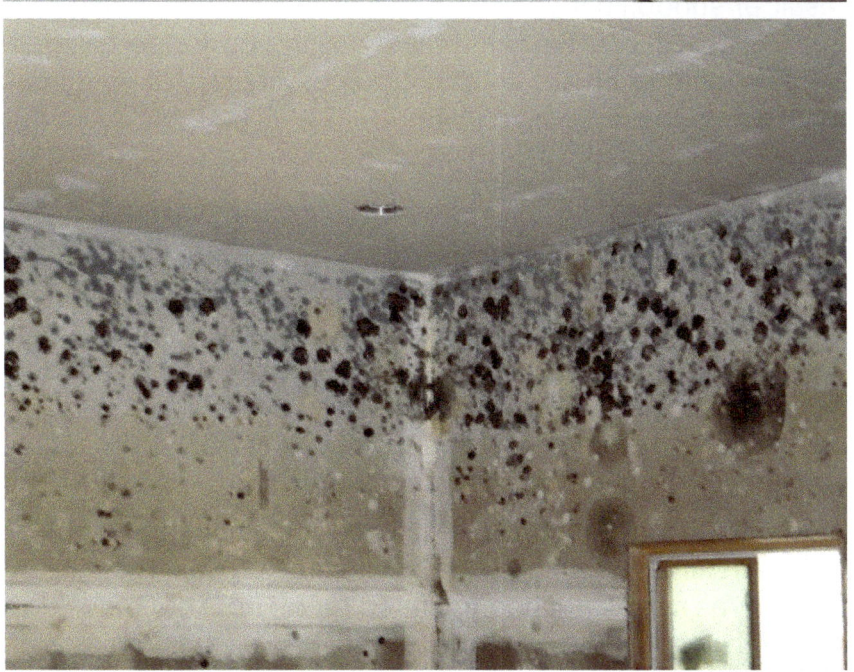

Heavy Metals, Carcinogens, PFAs, Phthalates & Pesticides and other Nasty chemicals (Tier 1)

One of the unfortunate costs of living in the modern world is dealing with all the different kinds of toxins humanity releases into the environment. It would be best to always avoid all types of pollution. Most of them are common sense; however, several can fly under the radar and cause long-term health issues that aren't easily noticeable straight away.

These pose a health risk to everybody. Healthy people will fare better but are greatly affected by these toxins. The effects on people recovering from a persistent virus can be devastating.

It's a sad reality that many modern chronic health issues can be attributed to these compounds. In many cases, they are the result of suboptimal choices made in our manufacturing and farming processes. Slowly, we are waking up to the damage we are doing to ourselves and our ecosystems. Do your best to eliminate these from your life.

Heavy Metals

It's been proven consuming foods with heavy metals is toxic to the brain and body. Ongoing exposure has been linked to low energy levels, damage to vital organs, and even Cancer. What hasn't been proven is how persistent viruses use the body's weakened state to reassert themselves. Mercury, Aluminum, Lead, and Cadmium can be found in some foods, polluted environments, and various everyday products.

One of the most unknown but increasingly common forms of heavy metal absorption is from contaminated seafood. Unfortunately, as more and more polluted runoff from our industries makes its way into the water systems, fish are being exposed to more heavy metals every year. The heavy metals are then passed back to us by eating cheap low-quality seafood. The primary nutritional reason for consuming seafood is the omega-3 content, as every other benefit can be sourced from either plants or land animals. Consuming seafood now and then won't cause too much trouble, especially if it's high quality and certified fresh, but I'd recommend eating no more than two serves every week.

Carcinogens

There are plenty of carcinogens that we can be exposed to in the modern world. Some of the most common are from pollution, car exhaust fumes, formaldehyde, and tobacco. Most of these are absorbed through our lungs as we breathe, which makes it difficult to avoid if you work in an industrial environment. Many household cleaning products are highly carcinogenic to touch and breathe in, such as bleach. If you suspect you're about to breathe some of this bad stuff in, either avoid the area altogether or put on a mask with a carbon filter.

In my early 20's I worked as a car mechanic at a Mazda dealership. The workshop I worked at had good ventilation fans, so I was lucky there, but there was no escaping the inevitable daily exposure. Surrounded by car fumes, dirty oils, greasy bearings, and petrol, I was repeatedly exposed to dangerous carcinogens. Luckily, I decided to change careers while I was still young, possibly avoiding many health problems later in life.

Another thing to watch out for is volatile organic compounds (VOC's) that are emitted from fresh products such as cars, furniture, paint, and pretty much anything that has that wonderful "new" smell. I once bought a couch that had that a strong new smell. It didn't bother me at first, but as the weeks went on my energy levels and focus were getting terrible. I did some research and found that the VOC's from the chemicals they used to treat the couch were slowly being emitted into the air I was breathing through a process called "off-gassing".

In some cases, the off-gassing can take quite a while or be particularly toxic. The best way to speed the off-gassing process is to put your new item out in the sun, making sure it's in a well-ventilated area. Do this for as long as it takes to remove the smell. It's easy with small handheld items but difficult with big bulky items like a couch. Consider buying secondhand furniture with minimal use if this is a problem for you, too.

PFA's

PFA's (per and polyfluoroalkyl's) are a group of man-made chemicals that have been used in household products for decades. Commonly found in non-stick cookware, the appeal to use them in frying pans comes from their strong chemical bond that repels water and oil. Due to this strength, PFA's don't decay in nature, and are transferred from the cookware we use to our food. Since they cannot be broken down, they stay in our bodies, disrupting the endocrine system (our hormone system) and placing a heavy burden on our natural detoxication systems.

Every single non-stick cooking pan that I've bought has eventually deteriorated and lost all its "non-stickiness". There have been all sorts of marketing attempts over the years to trick people to come back to them, such as stone-blasted pans or Teflon-coated pans. They always claim to be the ultimate fry pan that will never lose its non-stick coating, but each one of them does. The heat combined with the fats and proteins disrupts the coating, mixing in with your food.

The best alternatives to non-stick cookware are cast iron and stainless-steel fry pans. Cast iron is great for searing meats and cooking at high temperatures, but the pans can be heavy and require "seasoning" after each use. The seasoning process is wiping a thin layer of oil all over the fry pan to prevent oxidation (rust).

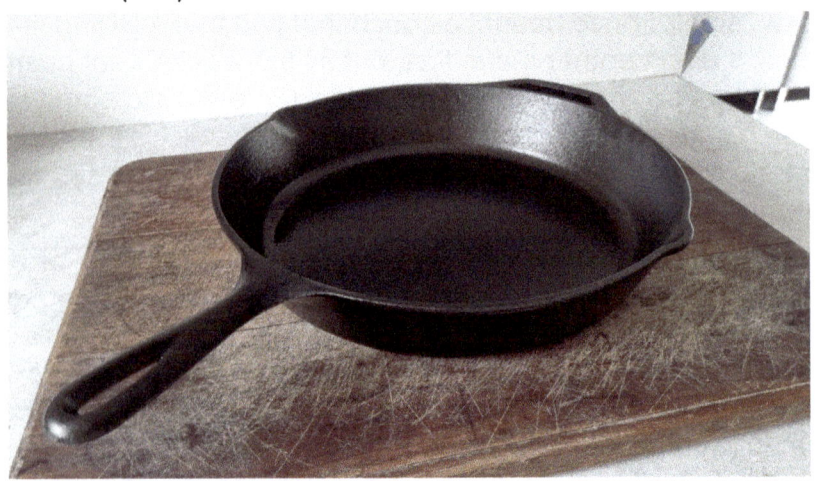

Stainless steel is better for everyday use. You can use it for stir fries and general meals. It's better to cook at medium temperatures with stainless steel as food can stick quite easily to it as temperatures rise.

If you can't give up the convenience of non-stick fry pans, there is one thing you need to remember. The higher the heat setting, the more the PFA's will degrade and leech into your food. Avoid cooking food with non-stick cookware past the medium heat setting.

Phthalates

Phthalates are a family of chemical compounds that are used in plastics to make them flexible and durable. They are also used in personal care products such as shampoos, soaps, and fragrances.

Society is just starting to take note of how these compounds are influencing our bodies. Phthalates interfere with our endocrine system by blocking the natural release of hormones, leading to a range of health issues, such as developmental and reproductive problems in both men and women.

Dr Shanna Swan wrote a book about how phthalate exposure in everyday products is threatening sperm count, altering sperm production in men and the menstrual cycle in women. Phthalates have also been linked to increasing the risk of developing obesity, diabetes, and cancer.

Here are some things to avoid to reduce Phthalate exposure:
- Plastic containers
- Plastic packaging
- Shampoos and Soaps that contain Phthalates

Many home maker stores are starting to stock glass food containers at reasonable prices. They might be a little heavier and require extra care, but for the on-going health benefits, they certainly are worth it.

Deodorants, Fragrances and Cleaning Products

Many household products such as cleaning agents, deodorants, fragrances and nail polish have dangerous chemicals in them that can be absorbed through the skin and by inhalation. These disrupt the immune system and place further burdens on the liver and lymphatic system.

In today's modern world, it's virtually impossible to avoid these completely. You can opt for natural products that aren't made with questionable chemicals, though these aren't as widely available and sometimes not as effective.

My favourite brand of deodorant decided to stop making their signature deodorant product, which I had grown quite attached to. It had no nasty chemicals in it, no side effects, smelled great, and lasted all day no matter what I did. I tried several others, but they either made me feel weird or just weren't very good at their job.

I later learned that several other supermarkets a few suburbs over had leftover stock of my favourite deodorant. I jumped in my car, drove to the nearest store, proceeded to the deodorant section, and loaded up on every single stick on the shelf (in total, about 12). At the time of writing, I'm about halfway through my supply, so I'm going to have to figure something new out eventually. But until that day, I'll stick with what works.

Another product which I've had issues with is cleaning sprays. There have been times when I've used a mould killing spray without a mask. This has always made me lightheaded and woozy afterwards, a classic sign of the liver being overburdened from breathing in the harmful chemicals.

If you're using a cleaning spray, make sure you've opened all your doors and windows to allow for maximum ventilation. A painter's mask will prevent you from breathing in any toxic fumes, and wearing high-quality rubber gloves will keep your skin safe.

As for deodorant, avoid products containing the following:
- Aluminum compounds
- Parabens
- Triclosan

For Fragrances/Perfumes, avoid those with:
- Synthetic musk's
- Formaldehyde
- Acetone
- Benzene

Pesticides

Last but not least are pesticides sprayed onto fruits and vegetables. You've probably heard of organic produce before. The difference between organic and non-organic produce often comes down to how it's farmed and what kind of soil it's grown in. The non-organic produce is planted in soil that has been fertilised with synthetic fertiliser, adding only a handful of minerals back into the soil. Organic produce is grown in naturally fertilised soil, giving the plants a much wider variety of natural minerals and microbes to grow from.

As vegetables and fruits grow, organic produce is not sprayed with pesticides to maintain crop yield, whereas non-organic produce commonly is. This prevents pests from feeding on the fruits and vegetables as they're growing, increasing the bottom lines for the farming companies. All food that gets shipped to market goes through a basic cleaning process, but this only focuses on the aesthetics of the produce and isn't concerned about any chemical residue left over.

You'll notice when eating organic food that it tends to have a stronger taste. Strawberries are a classic example; organic strawberries have a beautiful, sweet taste, but the non-organic stuff tastes dull and is almost like eating strawberry-flavoured cardboard.

If you are strapped for cash and can't justify buying organic produce, washing your fruits and vegetables is recommended. Not all need a wash; some come with their own protective layer (the outside skin), which can be peeled off. Fruits like bananas, oranges, and avocadoes have an outside skin that isn't consumed. Vegetables like carrots, onions, and potatoes require peeling their skin off and are generally safe. Every fruit or vegetable you eat with its outer layer intact will need a wash in warm water to remove the harmful chemicals. You can use bicarbonate soda or baking soda to go the extra mile.

Our bodies evolved to have many natural detoxication processes. Otherwise, the story of humanity would've ended a long time ago. The problem is the foods that nourished us in the past have changed as society has progressed. Modern farming techniques are lowering the nutritional content of our foods and are slowly exposing our bodies to more and more chemicals. This has a cumulative effect, where, at first, it's hardly noticeable, but decades later, mysterious problems start to arise.

The more toxins you can remove from your life, the less burden there will be on your body to do the extra work. Leaving more energy for the immune system and repairing organs.

Substance	Harmful Effects	Common Sources
Formaldehyde	- Respiratory irritation - Skin irritation - Carcinogenic potential	- Building materials (plywood, adhesives) - Some cosmetics, personal care products - Tobacco smoke
Acetone	- Eye, nose, and throat irritation - Central nervous system effects	- Nail polish remover - Paint thinners
Phthalates	- Endocrine disruption - Reproductive toxicity	- Plastic products (toys, food packaging) - Personal care products (fragrances)

Substance	Harmful Effects	Common Sources
Parabens	- Hormone disruption - Allergic reactions	- Cosmetics, skincare products
Aluminium	- Neurotoxicity - Linked to Alzheimer's	- Antiperspirants - Cookware, baking powder
Triclosan	- Endocrine disruption - Environmental impact	- Antibacterial soaps, toothpaste
Pesticides	- Neurological and developmental effects	- Conventionally grown fruits and veggies - Contaminated water
Heavy Metals	- Neurological damage - Kidney and liver damage	- Contaminated water, fish - Industrial pollution, some cosmetics
PFA's	- Developmental effects - Immune system effects	- Non-stick cookware, waterproof clothing - Stain-resistant fabrics, firefighting foam
Synthetic Fragrances	- Respiratory irritation - Allergic reactions	- Perfumes, colognes - Air fresheners, personal care products
Bisphenol A (BPA)	- Endocrine disruption - Reproductive issues	- Plastic containers, canned food linings
Glyphosate	- Potential carcinogen - Environmental impact - Potential carcinogen	- Herbicides (e.g., Roundup)

For more information about the toxins in our environment and food, I recommend reading any of Anthony William's books. He can be found at the following website:
https://www.medicalmedium.com/

Tap Water (Tier 1)

The quality of municipal tap water around the world varies greatly. It is never recommended to drink tap water in developing countries, and in many developed countries, chlorine is used to disinfect the water from pathogens. The information available about how tap water is treated can also vary. Some countries will have this information online, while other countries may not even have a water treatment program.

Each country (and even state) will have their own policy on how they treat their tap water. Generally, municipal water in developed countries is filtered quite well, getting rid of all the harmful pathogens and dirt particles through a complex filtration and disinfection system. While considered safe to drink by many authorities, there have been numerous studies showing drinking chlorinated water is detrimental to the body. Chlorine, even in low amounts, disrupts the endocrine system, downregulates important hormones, and raises inflammation.

Another common additive governments include in tap water is fluoride. Fluoride is commonly put in toothpaste and mouthwash with the intention to kill bacteria and create a barrier on your teeth so the enamel can grow. There have been many studies done proving topical fluoride has its benefits for teeth, however ingested fluoride is a different story.

Have you ever been to the dentist and had them apply a pasty substance to your teeth, which you've had to swish around in your mouth and spit out? That's a topical fluoride treatment. When you take a sip of water, do you swish it around your mouth for 30 seconds before swallowing? I certainly don't. It's been proven in a multitude of studies that ingested fluoride has no benefits to dental health. On-going consumption of fluoride has been shown to lower IQ, disrupt the thyroid, and excessive consumption leads to teeth discoloration.

Besides these two chemicals that are added in the treatment process, tap water must travel through sometimes hundreds of kilometers of metal pipes to get to your house. Unmaintained water pipes can cause metallic particles to leech into the water, creating further health issues. While the chance of this happening in developed countries is lower, it is difficult to guarantee that any water delivery system is 100% clean and safe.

The trouble with detecting poor quality water is that it requires expensive analysis equipment. However, someone who is quite perceptive and is used to drinking exceptional water will be able to tell if the water they are drinking is of average quality. Chlorinated and fluoridated water will not poison you, but they will impede your recovery ceiling and have a cumulative effect on your health over your life.

At the very minimum, I recommend drinking water from a water filter pitcher. These typically use a carbon filter that eliminates most of the chlorine and heavy metals in the water. To remove the fluoride, you'll need to spend a little bit more money. Reverse osmosis water filters in the past were the only solution for fluoride removal, but there are companies now selling bench top water filters that can remove fluoride too.

I've recently purchased a water filter that removes chlorine, fluoride, heavy metals, and just about everything else you wouldn't want to be drinking that's found in tap water. I can remember taking my first sip of it, and no joke, it felt like it was the first time I was drinking real water!

The purpose behind drinking filtered, mineralised, and alkalized water is that it is as close as possible to drinking natural spring water. Spring water is sourced from underground springs, where water filters through layers of rock and soil, removing impurities and adding minerals such as calcium, magnesium, and potassium. Many bottled water companies will advertise their water is from natural springs. However, they are often required to filter the water themselves to ensure its safety, and some companies simply filter municipal water themselves.

While sourcing your water from natural underground springs is likely unfeasible for most people, purchasing a high-quality water filter is affordable and pays dividends for your health.

Some of the things I noticed about myself after drinking water from a high-quality filter were:

- I feel clearer and less inflamed
- My emotions are smoother, and I have greater control over them
- My thoughts and ideas flow much better
- My voice has become stronger and resonates much clearer
- I have more energy and recover from exertion faster

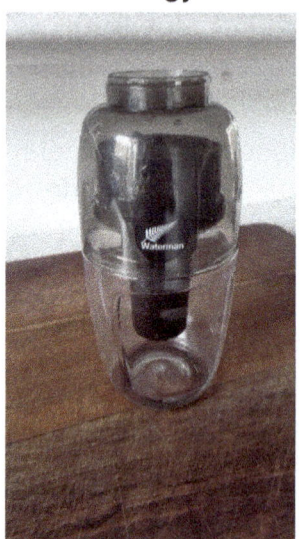

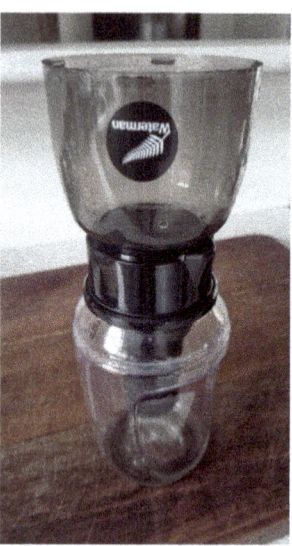

Eggs (Tier 2)

A critical food to stop consuming is eggs in any way, shape, or form. This was a big one for me to learn and implement into my life. Many years ago, I had begun my strength and fitness journey, and a friend had recommended I eat three eggs for breakfast every day. It was a revelation. I was stronger, felt better, and could push myself more in my professional and personal life. Unwittingly, when I got infected with EBV, I continued to eat three eggs for every breakfast, which I attribute as one of the biggest reasons why my recovery from EBV took so long.

It wasn't until I came across Anthony William and his book about thyroid healing that I found this crucial bit of information. He theorizes that eggs have an enormous number of hormones inside them for the chicken embryos to grow. In a healthy person, these hormones help with our energy production, strength, and even contribute to regulating our own hormones. However, in a person with an active viral infection, an egg with all its hormones acts as food for the virus to replicate on a large scale.

Another theory is that eggs have moderately high amount of histamine in them. Consuming them agitates the mast cells in your body and increases inflammation.

I'll be the first person to say, as a food, eggs are awesome. High in bio-available protein, good fats, nearly every vitamin and mineral you need, and if organically sourced, a good omega 3-6 profile. They're so versatile and make for a rocking ketogenic breakfast. I absolutely adore eggs, so it pains me greatly to tell you that when recovering from long-haul viral symptoms, they must be avoided.

Another thing to note is the prevalence of eggs in so many kinds of foods. Eggs are a great binding agent, used for baked goods, mayonnaise, salad dressings, sauces, and gravies. They are also very common in dessert foods, such as ice-cream, cakes, custard, pudding, meringue, tiramisu, and souffle. While it can be hard to resist such delicious treats, there are plenty of other alternatives that you can indulge in as you make progress with your recovery.

Something I noticed while I was consuming eggs after getting sick was I would have a tender "full" sensation under my left ribcage, right about where the spleen is. It felt like a lot of blood being focused there, and I had to be careful not to over-exert myself, or I'd experience a sharp pain in the area. When I stopped eating eggs, that sensation went away. Only to return to a smaller degree if I failed to avoid any other roadblocks on this list.

I stopped eating eggs for three months to really test the idea out. Curious to see if they still had an effect on me, I decided to fry up some eggs for breakfast one morning. I wasn't as debilitated by them, so there had been some progress, but that familiar sensation under my left ribcage came back for a few hours.

It was a big sacrifice for me to give up eggs. After all, they'd helped me so much as a go-to breakfast and a highly nutritious protein source. But after some time with their absence from my diet, I noticed my energy levels were higher, my capacity for work increased, and overall, I felt better. The ceiling on my recovery had lifted by a noticeable amount. But as time went on, I learned there was more I needed to do.

Eggs should always be avoided when recovering from a persistent virus.

Dairy Products (Tier 2)

After giving up eggs, I had to find something else to fill that gap in my breakfast. I knew it had to be a protein source, but the idea of eating something like beef in the morning was always a bit too heavy for me. I went to the supplement store and got myself a big tub of protein powder consisting entirely of the milk proteins, Whey, and Casein. Now, this alternative was pretty good; it gave me a similar kind of "boost" in the morning as eggs did, but without the fatigue and brain fog. At the time, I was still a student, so it was a cheap and easy way of consuming protein in the morning.

I managed to keep this up for a few years. It helped me finish my degree, get a job in my field, and begin my career as a Town Planner. But there was always a lingering feeling of the virus lurking in my body. I had to be careful not to push things too far, or else I'd be out of action for a long period of time. Essentially, the ceiling of my recovery had lifted, but it was still there. It wasn't until I got Covid, and my recovery was taking much longer than I expected, that I realised I had to make a change. I remember coming back to sport three weeks after the acute Covid phase, only to have my lungs in agony after a few minutes of moderate exertion. For months, it felt like my right lung had atrophied and wasn't working anymore. Any sort of deep breathing would hurt, and my sinuses were inflamed.

I eventually made the switch to chicken breast for breakfast as my protein source. This required a lot more planning for preparation, but it was worth it. Eventually, my energy returned, and my lungs got better. The ceiling had been raised again.

An important thing to consider when giving up dairy products is figuring out an alternative source of Calcium. The western world has been conditioned since the 1950's that cow's milk is the best way to get your RDI of Calcium every day. It's true dairy is a great source of Calcium. However, there are plenty of other ways to get it without poisoning yourself. Some of my favourites are:

- Almonds/Chia Seeds

    Tasty and nutritious, Almonds and Chia Seeds contain a high amount of Calcium. Just be careful not to consume too many, as they are high in calories.

- Broccoli

    Another great source of Calcium that has many other benefits too. I'd recommend eating Broccoli as much as you can throughout the week.

- Kale/Leafy Greens

    Kale has the highest content of Calcium among the leafy greens. It also has the most impressive nutrient profile among them. Just be careful not to have it all the time, as it can disrupt Thyroid function. Spinach is also a good alternative.

- Beans and Lentils

    Whites Beans, Navy Beans, and Lentils are all good sources of non-dairy Calcium. They also contain complex unprocessed carbohydrates, B-Vitamins and several other vitamins we need.

- Fortified Plant Milks

    Many plant milks such as Almond, Oat, and Cashew milk are artificially fortified with Calcium. While better than nothing, these are rarely absorbed well and shouldn't be a person's only source of Calcium.

- Marine Sourced Calcium

    There are marine plants very high in Calcium. These can be found in supplement form for easy consumption and are the only form of Calcium I recommend in a capsule. Google marine sourced Calcium to find a brand you like.

Dairy in the form of high-quality **grass-fed & finished cheese and butter** is acceptable in small amounts when recovering from a persistent virus. The higher quality of the source, the less impact it will have on your immune system. Cow's milk from supermarkets is 99% of the time pasteurized and homogenised to the point where any of the natural benefits that may offset the downsides are completely neutralised. I would recommend removing cow's milk from your diet altogether, even for a healthy person. Whey and Casein protein powders should be avoided while recovering too.

Added Sugars, Processed Foods, and Artificial Sweeteners (Tier 2)

These are really no brainers. It's becoming common knowledge that refined sugar and processed foods make you fat, unhealthy, and age you prematurely. Our bodies just weren't designed to process these artificial products in any kind of healthy way.

When recovering from chronic viral symptoms, it's even more important to steer clear of these foods. Not only will they impair your basic metabolic functions, but they also contribute to feeding the virus. Actively regressing your progress.

Consuming processed, refined sugar triggers a sharp Insulin response (the hormone our bodies produce to move sugar from our blood to our cells). In a healthy person, they experience a "sugar rush". But as we age, our metabolism slows, and our insulin response isn't as effective as it used to be, meaning we need more Insulin to respond to the sugar in our blood.

Think of sugar as a dangerous addictive drug. The first few times you take it, it's not so bad, and you feel great, especially when you're young. I remember when I was a teenager, I used to come home from a shift at work and drink a can of Pepsi while eating a full block of white chocolate. These days that kind of indulgence would make me sick, only reserved for special occasions, followed by a period of long fasting to reset my metabolism.

The problem with sugar, like any kind of drug, is with repeated consumption, you become accustomed to how much you get, and you need more to get that same feeling. The more you eat, the greater damage you do to your ageing body. Not only that, but your ability to bounce back diminishes, too. Creating a downward spiral of devastation to your health.

An excess of Insulin leads to all sorts of metabolic diseases and stifles our immune system. For more information about the subject, Dr Berg on YouTube is the best source for concise summaries of the medical literature.

As you start to become more aware of what goes into processed packaged foods, you'll see that added sugar is in everything. Cereals, biscuits, "healthy" bars, fruit juice, and bread are instilled with added sugar to preserve their shelf life and make them taste good.

To process these added sugars, our bodies reprioritize B-Vitamins, Vitamin C, and Zinc to deal with the inflammation and stress they place on our energy production system. So not only does sugar make you fat, but it also makes your immune system weaker!

Many people think they can get around the sugar dilemma by drinking soft drinks with artificial sweeteners. These may have no sugar in them, but artificial sweeteners have been proven to raise the insulin response just as high as a comparable amount of sugar does. The clue is in their name, "artificial". Again, our bodies don't know how to process these synthetic additives. I once tried switching over to Diet Pepsi to see if it was a viable alternative. I hated how it tasted and found I felt even worse after consuming it. There is literally no upside to consuming artificially sweetened drinks.

As I said earlier, I do enjoy a bit of a sugar binge from time to time. It all comes down to how you take care of yourself before the binge session. If for 90% of the time, you are watching what you are eating, and 10% of the time, you splurge out, it's not going to be a big deal. The body can handle the odd disruption, but what you do every day is what counts.

Bear in mind if you are suffering severe viral symptoms or dealing with metabolic issues, then I would recommend giving up sugar for as long as you can. Until you can return to moderate exercise (which is excellent at improving the insulin response), sugar should be off the menu.

Vegetable & Seed Oils (Tier 2)

When most people think of a vegetable, they think of something that is healthy and nutritious. Unfortunately, the majority of oils extracted from vegetables are highly processed and chemically altered for mass production and preservation. Some examples you've probably heard of are:

- Canola oil
- Soybean oil
- Corn oil
- Sunflower oil
- Safflower oil
- Cottonseed oil

These are all incredibly inflammatory to the body and can be found everywhere in processed packaged food.

The trouble starts with their levels of omega-6 fatty acids. While it is true we need some omega 6, it needs to be in balance with omega 3s, optimally a ratio of 1:3 or lower omega 3 to 6 fatty acids. Vegetables and seed oils have vastly skewed ratios of omega 6. The problem is these vegetable oils are everywhere in processed food, take away, and even low-quality restaurant meals. If you look at the ingredients of nearly any packaged product, you'll see there is some form of vegetable or seed oil present.

Pre-prepared vegan food is notoriously high in these kinds of oils. Many people think they are choosing the healthy option when something in a package says "Vegan". Sadly, many companies use these low-quality oils with artificial additives and sugar to increase their profit margins, desirability, and shelf life. They might not have any animal products in them, but they are far from healthy.

High-Intensity Exercise and High Adrenaline Activities (Tier 2)

Another love of mine. For a healthy person, high-intensity exercises are great for fitness and general conditioning. They stimulate fat burning, activate fast twitch muscles, and release high levels of growth hormone into the bloodstream. However, for a person recovering from a persistent virus, they're hazardous to the healing process. Put simply, the quick release of adrenaline startles the immune system and doesn't give it a chance to respond to the increase in stress. As discussed earlier, EBV affects the lymphatic system and any kind of sharp change in blood pressure puts a high load on the pumping mechanism to the lymph nodes. Normally, this isn't a problem, but for someone with a persistent virus, this will overstress the lymphatic system nodes and reactivate the virus.

Other viruses that cause long-haul symptoms are similar in this regard. Typically, when engaging in high intensity activities, our bodies need a lot of oxygen to keep our muscles functioning. Covid primarily affects the lungs and their ability to absorb oxygen into the bloodstream. Forcing your lungs to work extra hard before they've recovered will only make things worse. Not only will it be stunting your recovery, but also increasing the risk of developing scar tissue throughout the lungs.

Besides the intense inflammation high intensity exercises produce, the immune system is turned off by the rapid uptake of adrenaline in the blood, giving the virus free reign to propagate itself and infect more cells. What's more, high intensity exercise turns on what's called the after-burner effect and keeps your body in slightly elevated stress state for up to 2 days. This is a great sales pitch for a fat-burning course, but for anyone recovering from a persistent virus, is not good news.

Clearly, if you're suffering from severe long covid, any kind of activity will be difficult for you. This advice is primarily for those with mild to moderate symptoms, who think they can come back to their old lifestyle straight away. With enough time and patience, you will be able to do the things you used to be able to. It just takes time to heal and build yourself back up.

For me, working out at a high level of intensity was like therapy. I could always rely on going out on my bike and giving myself a thrashing to clear my head. There were several occasions where I thought I could push past my limits when I was recovering. But every time I did, I'd always find myself crashing hard for the next few days, falling behind in my studies or daily duties.

I hate to say it, but you need to withdraw from these activities for a good amount of time. I've got plenty of alternative activities in the next chapter, but understand that while you may be itching to get back out there and go hard like you used to, it's vital to take it easy for a while.

Moderate Steady State Cardio/Endurance Activities (Tier 2)

For all the runners out there, I'm afraid to say you'll need to take a break from those epic treks you may have previously enjoyed. Even with a moderate pace, any kind of exertion for extended periods will overtax your adrenals. I know you've probably got the attitude of "no pain, no gain" in your head, which is normally a good thing. But when you're recovering, pushing yourself is always a bad idea.

You need to find a kind of exercise that gets you moving in a gentle way. When I was recovering from EBV, I had to stop all HIIT and strength training for a while. Walking was just about all I could do, and eventually, I slowly came back to cycling.

Exercise of any kind is a tax on your adrenal glands. Doing too much will raise adrenaline and cortisol, the two hormones you need to steer clear of while recovering. This comes back to the ceiling principle, when you are recovering, you cannot exceed the ceiling in any kind of activity, or you will face an unpleasant crash.

After catching Covid, which turned into Long-Covid, my lung capacity was greatly reduced, and any kind of aerobic exercise longer than 5 minutes would place too much stress on my lungs. I could do moderate strength training and even some interval training as long as I gave my lungs repeated breaks.

Aerobic exercise will help to improve your recovery, but the key is to find the optimal range of intensity you can handle. You don't need to do too much to stay healthy, try and work up to 20 minutes each day of light exercise to stay healthy and sane.

Moderate to Heavy Weight Training (Tier 2)

This won't apply to everyone, but for those who enjoy chasing gains at the gym, you're going have to wind it back for a while.

Like the last two points, I had a hard time letting go of this too. Pushing myself to build muscle and strength has always been incredibly satisfying. After several months of rest, I was ready to get back out there and work on my progress. Sadly, it was the same kind of story of the last two activities. The intense lifting places a heavy burden on your adrenals, increasing inflammation and diverts precious resources away from your immune system to repairing your muscles.

All kinds of moderate to heavy lifting must be avoided for a while. When you start to feel better, try lifting very light weights at high reps and see how it feels. You'll want a weight you can do at least 25 reps without placing too much strain on yourself. The idea here is to exercise for the health benefits like better circulation and lymphatic drainage, not to get stronger or build muscle. With time, you'll slowly get stronger.

Alcohol (Tier 2)

This can be a tough one, especially for young people. Alcohol impairs your immune system by making your body focus on processing the alcohol that's coming in. Many popular alcoholic drinks are paired up with sugary soft drinks, a double whammy for holding back your immune system.

The obvious answer is to stop drinking all kinds of alcoholic drinks entirely. There have been many studies done that demonstrate any alcohol consumption is detrimental to your health; it is a poison, after all. However, I know there are those out there who also think life is too short to refrain from the occasional indulgence every now and then.

Since everyone has different tolerances, it's difficult to give a clear recommendation. Being from Australia, I know how hard it is to avoid alcohol sometimes. But what I do know for sure is that it should be avoided for at least three months after the initial infection. From then, you can test the waters with perhaps two standard drinks. You'll need to wait **6 months MINIMUM** of consistent progress before you can even consider more than that. Trust me, if you haven't recovered properly, you won't even enjoy yourself, and the hangover will be like nothing you've ever experienced.

I know many cultures around the world enjoy alcohol from time to time. So, if you're starting to feel better and are returning to normal activities, a glass or two won't throw you back very far. But whatever you do, avoid **binge drinking**.

Illegal Drugs (Tier 2)

Obvious to some, but not always to others, most illegal drugs either raise adrenaline or suppress the immune system. The body must work hard to flush these substances out of a healthy person. You can imagine the implications for a person fighting off a persistent virus who takes illegal drugs.

There are some drugs out there that act as a... "relaxant" on the body. I don't condone taking any kind of drug unless it's necessary as an anti-viral or anti-inflammatory, but there certainly are some out there that have less of an impact on the body. In terms of recovering from a persistent virus, in theory, these could help keep anxiety and stress under control. You'll need to use your discretion and trust that you'll have the awareness to make the right call for yourself.

Processed Grains/Flour Products (Tier 3)

The next item in the litany of man-made foods are processed grain and flour products. I've said to **limit** your consumption of processed grain and flour products because in the modern world, eliminating them from your diet is nigh impossible for the average person. Foods like Pasta, Sandwiches, and Burgers are engrained into our culture as food we share with friends or family. They aren't going to actively make you sick, but consuming them regularly will raise inflammation and make it harder for your immune system to do its job.

As I stated previously, the body uses B-Vitamins and Zinc to digest and convert these foods into energy. So, you may be getting some easy calories in, but reducing the nutritional resources your immune system needs to fight the virus.

Many breads and cereals are "fortified" with synthetic B-Vitamins to stop this problem. These can be considered slightly better, but still will be of a net negative to your health.

Just about anything that comes in a packet has been processed for maximum shelf life and taste. You might feel satiated, but eating processed grains and flour will bring you down slowly.

The best alternatives to processed carbohydrates are the unprocessed natural kind:

- All kinds of Potatoes (Sweet Potatoes are great)
- Legumes (Lentils, Beans and Chickpeas)
- Brown and Black Rice
- Fruit

Lower stress from finances, relationships, and work (Tier 3)

By now, you're probably starting to understand that all kinds of stress take a toll on the body. It's true; we need some stress to keep us moving forward. The daily struggles of work, relationships, and finances are fine for a healthy person, but for someone recovering, it can be too much of a burden. What you don't want to subject yourself to is chronic stress.

Chronic stress is defined as a consistent sense of feeling pressured or overwhelmed by outside factors. In a healthy person, the symptoms of chronic stress will likely show themselves as being moody, having poor focus, and low energy. In a person with a persistent virus, chronic stress can be debilitating and lead to a reactivation of symptoms from the acute phase of the infection. Chronic stress may be unavoidable from time to time, but in general, it's never good news. It depletes your adrenals, shrinks your thymus gland (part of the lymphatic system), and allows the virus to get ahead of the immune response.

Several months after I contracted EBV, I was given the opportunity to move out of home and live with a few friends. While nowhere near full recovery, I couldn't pass up the opportunity to get out of my parent's home and start living on my own terms. Initially, it was great fun; the freedom to live how I wanted was liberating. But I soon came to learn that one of my housemates really took a lot of energy away from me. I've always enjoyed a quiet, peaceful house, but this person just loved living life at full blast. They were in a rock band, and our personalities clashed.

Slowly but surely, living with this person took a toll on my mental health and wore me down. I spoke with the other housemate, who I was much closer with about them, and we all had a sit down one night to discuss some of the issues. Even with a bit of a chat, things didn't get much better. I realised the only way I'd alleviate the stress was to get out of there and move back to my parents' house. The chronic stress was not worth it to live on my own terms.

Depending on your level of recovery, acute stress can be managed if it's within reasonable limits and enough time is given so your adrenals can be replenished. I found that once I got to a certain level of recovery, I could push myself for a day or two, providing I knew I'd have plenty of time to take it easy afterward.

For an optimal recovery, you want to remove as many burdens from your life as possible.

Caffeine (Tier 3)

Caffeine essentially works by putting the body into a stressed state. This gives you that pleasant perky buzz by releasing adrenaline, raising cortisol, and blocking the adenosine receptors in your brain, which are responsible for making you tired. All of this makes your adrenals work harder. There are a few cognitive changes that occur too, but in terms of immunity, caffeine suppress recovery in favour of performance right now.

Not everyone is affected by caffeine in the same way. This is why there are people who can drink multiple cups a day right up until the evening and don't have any trouble sleeping. For others like me, it's like having anxiety, but faster. Overall, I would give up caffeine for the acute infection recovery, and if you are more susceptible to it, maybe hold off for several months.

CHAPTER SUMMARY: WHAT TO STOP DOING

Stop consuming these foods:

1. Stop consuming MSG-laden foods (Tier 1)
   - Toxic to the brain and disrupts hormones
2. Stop eating eggs (Tier 2)
   - They feed viruses and encourage a histamine response
3. Stop consuming dairy products (Tier 2)
   - They feed viruses and clog up your lymphatic system
4. Stop consuming processed foods with added sugar and artificial sweeteners (Tier 2)
   - Messes with your hormones and burdens your liver
5. Stop consuming foods with vegetable and seed oil in them (Tier 2)
   - Highly inflammatory and disrupt your endocrine system
   - Makes sunburn more common
6. Limit processed grain/flour products (Tier 3)
   - Promotes inflammation in the digestive system, bad for hormones.

Stop doing these activities:

1. Stop doing high intensity sports, exercise, or anything that raises adrenaline (Tier 2)
    - Adrenaline turns off your immune system and raises inflammation
    - Depletes your adrenal glands
2. Stop doing moderate steady state cardiovascular exercise (Tier 2)
    - Raises inflammation and depletes your adrenal glands
3. Stop doing moderate to heavy weight training (Tier 2)
    - Places a high demand on your nervous system
    - Depletes adrenals and raises inflammation

Stop exposing yourself to these:

1. Stop exposing yourself to mould (Tier 1)
    - Highly toxic to humans and strips the immune system away
2. Stop drinking alcohol (Tier 2)
    - A toxin that must be processed by the liver
3. Stop smoking and vaping
    - Loaded with chemicals and carcinogens
4. Stop drinking caffeine (Tier 2)
    - Raises stress and overburdens the liver
5. Stop taking unhelpful drugs (Tier 2)
    - Disrupts hormones, burdens the liver, and impairs the immune system
6. Stop exposing yourself to heavy metals, PFA's, Phthalates, Pesticides, and other nasty chemicals (Tier 1)
    - Hormone disrupters and immune system damagers

7. Stop stressing out over money, relationships, and work (Tier 3)
    - Depletes adrenal glands and turns off the immune system
8. Stop drinking straight tap water and filter it (Tier 1)
    - Chlorine, fluoride, and other nasties will impair your immune system and hormones

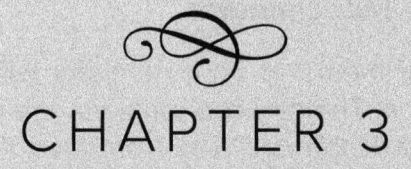

CHAPTER 3
TURBOCHARGE YOUR IMMUNE SYSTEM

This chapter will not be broken up into a tier list, as everything here is essential to helping your immune system fight off the virus and rebuild your body. It may be difficult to do everything on this list every day, so just try a few out and make them a daily habit before you get stuck into the rest. The improvements you see should give you a hunger for more results and a willingness to implement more changes.

Supporting the Mitochondria

The overarching theme to your recovery will be to support your mitochondria. The mitochondria are commonly known as the powerhouse of the cell. They produce ATP, the primary energy currency of the body, through a process called cellular respiration. I won't bore you with biology lesson, but suffice it to say if your mitochondria are dysfunctional, you won't have the energy to do anything. They are part of every cell in your body. Supporting their functionality is paramount.

As we discussed earlier in this book, the condition is highly complex and requires a holistic approach. However, addressing mitochondrial dysfunction is the key, as all roads lead back to it in some way.

- Lower oxidative stress - improve mitochondrial function
- Remove environmental toxins - improve mitochondrial function
- Fix chronic inflammation - improve mitochondrial function
- Cure infections - improve mitochondrial function

With every step you take in recovering, you will be supporting your mitochondria to produce more ATP, meaning more energy your cells can generate to give you back your life.

Covering all your nutritional bases

While there are vitamins and minerals that help the immune system more than others, a deficiency in any of them will influence your overall immunity and health. Without going into excruciating detail about each of them, suffice it to say, they have a synergistic role in keeping you alive and healthy. It's important all vitamins and minerals are present in your diet.

A key difference between some of the vitamins is how **soluble** they are in the body. Fat-soluble vitamins (A, D, E, and K) are absorbed with dietary fat and stored in the liver until they are needed by the body. Water soluble vitamins (B's and C) are absorbed directly into the bloodstream and are not stored to any significant extent.

The human body can load up on fat-soluble vitamins from one day of healthy eating; however, with water-soluble vitamins, any excess consumed does not stay in the body for long and is excreted through urine. Therefore, we need to be regularly consuming foods with these important vitamins in order to stay healthy.

The best way to make sure you are covering all nutritional bases is to use a food diary such as Cronometer. This is available for free online and with their app. It allows you to input all the food you've eaten in a day and lists all micro and macro nutrients found in those foods. With this data, it shows you how close you are to hitting the recommended daily intakes for all the standard nutritional requirements based on your age, sex, and body type.

Every meal having a vitamin C source

Vitamin C is a highly important vitamin for your immune system and other key parts of the body. It is used in several immune system processes, tissue repair, and adrenal support. Eating vegetables or fruit high in vitamin C with every meal is the best way to ensure your recovery never comes off the train tracks. As stated above, our bodies do not store this important vitamin. Meaning every 4 hours, what remains in our bloodstream is excreted through our urine. This is why, when recovering, having some kind of vitamin C source in every meal is so important.

Do not be tempted to buy a big bottle of "vitamin C" tablets from your local pharmacy. Chances are it's only "ascorbic acid" in tablet form, which gives you hardly any of the benefits of natural vitamin C. In the supplements chapter, I talk about natural vitamin C capsules, which are effective but should not replace natural food sources completely.

It is also notable that consuming high levels of sugar and carbohydrates causes our bodies to need more vitamin C. The cause of this has been theorized by Dr Shawn Baker who analyzed the molecular structure of both vitamin C and glucose, finding both molecules have a similar atomic structure. Leading to the theory that vitamin C competes with glucose for absorption in the body. When high levels of glucose are present in the bloodstream, less vitamin C is absorbed.

Nearly all fruits and vegetables have vitamin C in them. Salads are the best and easiest way to get your vitamin C fix because of how versatile they can be. Throw some leafy greens into a bowl, a few chopped tomatoes, avocado, extra virgin olive oil (EVOO), and some lime juice, and bam! You've got yourself a refreshing and cleansing salad loaded with natural vitamin C.

A compound found in extra virgin olive oil, hydroxytyrosol, was found in a study to aid in the absorption of vitamin C from food. Subjects in the control group experienced higher levels of blood plasma vitamin C levels compared to those in the placebo group. I would recommend adding EVOO to all your salads.

A great alternative to fresh fruits and vegetables is **sauerkraut**. Centuries ago, Sailors crossing the oceans for months rarely had access to any kind of fresh produce. You can imagine the kinds of foods that were kept for those long voyages weren't the most nutritionally dense. A common problem arose when sailors developed scurvy, a disease that produces symptoms such as bleeding gums, fatigue, and bruising all due to the deficiency in vitamin C.

As refrigeration was yet to be invented, they had to find some kind of vegetable that would keep on the long voyages. Alas, sauerkraut was chosen as it could be placed in brine at the start of the voyage and left to slowly ferment as the journey unfolded, allowing sailors to take out portions as needed.

Using Extra Virgin Olive Oil everywhere

In the Mediterranean, EVOO is a staple of their diet, where they use it for dipping bread with spices, cooking, and drizzling it over their pastas. It's widely agreed amongst the scientific community that people who consume a Mediterranean diet have consistently lower levels of inflammation and live longer lives. Besides the great living conditions and quality of vegetables available there, EVOO has been found in numerous studies to be a big part of health and longevity.

The primary nutrients found in EVOO:

- Vitamin E – a powerful antioxidant and critical vitamin we rarely get enough of
- Chlorophyll – the compound which makes plants green. Helps to clean out the blood
- Polyphenols – Compounds which have an antioxidant effect on the body
- Phytosterols – Help reduce vasculature inflammation
- Monounsaturated fats – A great energy source and anti-inflammatory

I must warn you that plenty of EVOO products sold in supermarkets are not what they seem. Many producers dilute their olive oil to increase profits, and some substitute it with seed oils mixed with beta carotene to give it the green/yellow colour. The real deal will taste almost grassy, with small particles flowing through the oil.

When I started using EVOO as my salad dressing, I noticed a considerable leap in my recovery. I had taken up eating a salad every day to kickstart my recovery but was using cheap salad dressings I bought from my supermarket to improve the taste.

I had a mental barrier; these processed salad dressings where the only way of dressing a salad. One day during a shop, I read the labels, and the ingredient lists on these products shocked me. Nearly all were loaded with seed oils, artificial ingredients, and sugar. I decided that sacrificing a little bit of taste by using plain EVOO was how I would continue to dress my salads.

Getting adequate Zinc from natural sources every day

Zinc is a mineral many people are deficient in. It performs many essential roles in our immune system, repairs tissue from damage, and is also required in almost 100 enzymes to carry out vital chemical reactions. Zinc was the first mineral I focused on when I got sick. Zinc is the most abundant in **red meats, seafood, and organs.** There are trace amounts in other foods, but without eating any of these regularly; it can be difficult to get enough zinc to keep the body healthy.

Something to consider when optimizing your zinc intake is whether other foods you are consuming contain high levels of phytic acid. Phytic acid is an anti-nutrient found in many grains and nuts that blocks the absorption of zinc. Providing you are getting sufficient levels of zinc in your diet, you don't need to worry about this too much, but the foods highest in phytic acid are as follows:

Grains: Wheat, Oats, Rice

Legumes: Beans, Peanuts and Lentils

Nuts and Seeds: Walnuts, Almonds and Pinenuts

Consuming any of these in low to moderate amounts will not have a big impact on your zinc levels if you are getting adequate levels of zinc from food. However, if your diet is devoid of food with easily absorbed zinc, you may need to consider other strategies for getting enough zinc such as:

Soaking: Soaking nuts in water overnight can reduce the phytic acid content

Fermentation: Fermenting foods can break down phytic acid and increase the bioavailability of zinc

Consume a high amount of quality vegetables

Eating a vegetable will never make your day worse. Unless you've just you've just taken a bite of an eggplant (kidding). Sure, they don't always taste the greatest, but they can be prepared in many ways that complement a meal. After getting into the habit of eating vegetables regularly, you'll enjoy the vitality boost they give you. They're loaded with vitamins, minerals and are naturally low in calories. Vegetables are a gift from nature that keep us strong and healthy.

It is worth noting that cooking any kind of vegetable within an inch of its life will neutralize many of the nutrients stored within. Some vegetables need more cooking than others to become palatable, but often, they only need a light sauté or steam.

Another note is some vegetables can be detrimental to your health when consumed in high amounts. Everyone reacts differently, but Kale can block thyroid hormones when consumed in large quantities regularly. Spinach contains oxalates that can create kidney stones, and many beans and nuts have phytic acid, which block zinc absorption. While it can be tedious to learn more about boring old vegetables, they can provide so much value to your life when added appropriately.

Raw carrots are great at detoxifying the gut of bad bacteria and fungal growth. They help the body to rebalance the GI microbiome in a gentle, non-invasive way. Plus, they're cheap and easy to eat raw. Just give them a good wash under water and allow them to dry naturally.

When I started eating raw carrots every day before breakfast, I noticed I didn't get my normal hunger cravings at about 10 am. Previously, I would have breakfast at 7 am, followed by a mid-morning meal of Oats and peanut butter to get me through to lunch. By eating one carrot before breakfast, I no longer had an energy crash at 10 am and could power on.

For people with severely disrupted gut microbiomes, it may take a few weeks to see any improvements, but rest assured, the carrots will be working hard to restore the good bacteria inside your gut.

For optimal recovery and health, I recommend eating 7-10 servings of vegetables every day. The easiest way to do this is by eating a **big salad** with lunch or dinner. In the recipes sections you'll find the kinds of salads I like to make.

Find a Greens Powder that works for you

If you're finding it hard to eat vegetables with every meal, then I recommend finding a high-quality Greens Powder that agrees with you. I've sampled several over the years and can report they are all slightly different in their nutritional profile and how they affect the body.

The most common ingredients in greens powders are Spirulina, wheatgrass powder, barley grass powder, and Chlorella. These are highly nutritious plants and contain many phytonutrients that aid the immune system, detoxification, and help to build your body back up.

When I say find one that works for you, I mean not every product on the market is high quality or will agree with you. The plants could've been sourced from bad conditions or processed in a way that kills many of the nutrients. Besides the cheapest products available, most will provide some level of nutritional value to you. If you can, I wouldn't waste time with the cheap stuff. You get what you pay for with Green Powders, and spending that bit extra will improve your energy and recovery significantly.

Besides being loaded with vitamins, minerals, and phytonutrients, they also raise your blood alkalinity, which lowers inflammation and prevents arterial damage. Any sort of plant that is green coloured will have chlorophyll, the pigment that gives it its green colour. Chlorophyll has massive benefits for the body, such as being an antioxidant, and detoxifying the liver and lymphatic system.

Whenever I feel an illness coming on, the first thing I do is make a smoothie with a few scoops of my favourite greens powder. Immediately after consuming, I feel my spirit rise, and a peaceful calm falls over me as I lie on my couch recuperating.

Having a high-quality greens powder in my routine has been paramount to my recovery.

While you're recovering, stick with Chicken and Beef

This advice is important to everyone, not just the athletes and bodybuilders. You need protein to build your body back up. Protein isn't just for muscles; it's used for countless functions in the body and is necessary to rebuild internal organs and tissue.

As discussed earlier, eggs and dairy are off the menu. I know they're some of the cheapest and most accessible protein you can get, but while you're recovering, they cannot be consumed. Chicken breast is ideal as it's the cleanest of the animal meats. It's also a great protein source and has a respectable vitamin and mineral profile too.

Lean cuts of Beef are also very nutritious. They are rich in protein, B-Vitamins, contain heme Iron (much better absorbed by the body), omega 3's, and have high amounts of zinc. Not only that, beef tastes great. Just make sure you're buying quality grass-fed cuts of beef. The grain-fed animals are not nearly as nutritious.

While it's possible to get by without eating meat, it is very difficult to source all the essential vitamins, minerals, fatty acids, and proteins which are present in animal foods. It can be argued that a plant-based diet is cleaner for the body, but sticking with one for more than a week places too much risk of a protein and nutrient deficiency. Most plant sources of zinc have quite low levels of the mineral, to begin with and contain high levels of phytic acid. The protein from plants is also not a complete protein. It commonly is missing entire amino acids of a protein chain or contains much lower levels than animal sources.

It should be noted that if you are suffering from severe symptoms, you may need to focus on fruits and vegetables for a time until your body alkalizes enough to the point where you can consume animal products again. Animal meat does raise blood acidity levels and can be heavy to digest for those with burdened immune systems. If it feels like your body is starting to settle down, try to get high quality pasture raised/grass-fed animal products, as these won't increase inflammation on the same scale as the alternatives.

If you're a vegan, it is possible to supplement deficiencies in your diet, though it's important to get high-quality supplements that are absorbable. The key nutrients to focus on are protein, zinc, iron, vitamin B12, and omega 3s (DHA & EPA).

High-quality wild-caught fish is also a good choice, but with the levels of pollution and heavy metals leeching into the ocean, it's hard for me to recommend fish for recovery. If you can get high-quality seafood, I recommend Salmon, Sardines, and Oysters. They all contain great amounts of omega 3s, protein, selenium, zinc, calcium, and iodine. I've been finding the quality of the seafood in supermarkets has been dropping steadily over the last ten years. Supermarkets source much of their seafood from fish farms, where they can control the breeding process.

So far, the only source of high-quality seafood I've found has been from companies that send you a box of frozen meat direct to your door and quality fish markets supplied by local fishers. The product tends to be better, and more money goes to local producers.

Get at least 15 minutes of good sun exposure every day

The sun isn't just for tanning. When exposed to sunlight, human skin creates vitamin D, a natural immune booster and hormone regulator. Vitamin D is necessary for a significant amount of hormone and enzymatic functions in the body. It boosts well-being, immunity, and testosterone production in men. The best thing about Vitamin D is it's free! Providing you live in an area that gets decent sunlight throughout the year. I know, not everyone lives near the equator, and for most of winter, it can be hard to get adequate sun exposure. In these cases, supplementation is critical. Vitamin D is best absorbed in a capsule when it's in oil form.

Whenever I'm working at home during the day, and I'm feeling a bit stressed out or low on energy, I'll take out a Yoga mat and lie on the grass outside for 20 minutes. When I'm deficient in Vitamin D, I can almost instantly feel my body thanking me for the sun exposure. My muscles start to relax, my mind begins to clear, and my breathing slows and gets deeper. It practically puts me into a meditative state as I soak up my daily requirement for sun.

A little trick I learned from a YouTuber a while back is when it's best to get sun exposure. There are two types of ultraviolet radiation we receive, UVA and UVB. UVB is the type that creates vitamin D when it touches our skin. This occurs during the middle of the day when the sun is at its strongest. You can tell when it changes back to UVA by looking at the height of shadows. For example, if your shadow is shorter in length than your height, that indicates UVB is beaming down on you. Conversely, when shadows are longer than the height of objects that are casting them, UVA is shining down.

The amount of sun exposure necessary to produce healthy levels of Vitamin D will vary from person to person. Those with more pigmentation (darker skin) will absorb it slower but can stay outside longer before burning. Those with less pigmentation (lighter skin) will absorb it faster, but the risk of sunburn increases higher the longer you are exposed. Overall, I'd recommend 15-30 minutes of lying in the sun with your chest and legs exposed, scaling it up depending on your complexion. There are, of course, risks of sunburn if exposure exceeds these time frames, so be careful, and if spending longer than 30 minutes in the sun, apply sun protection after those 30 minutes. Sunscreen, while useful, does block the absorption through our skin.

Morning sun exposure when UVA is beaming down is great for hormonal priming and boosting your mood upon waking. I make a beeline to my backyard when I wake up and stand in the sun for 5 minutes. I've noticed my productivity, mood, and energy levels are much higher now that I've taken this practice up.

Bonus points if you take your shoes off and walk on grass barefoot while getting your sun exposure. There have been several new studies showing that "grounding" yourself by putting your skin to the ground, lowers inflammation and boosts your immune system and mood. Every time I go outside to the park, I whip my shoes off and walk around barefoot, taking great care not to step on anything sharp, of course. I feel noticeably calmer and more focused within about 10 minutes.

For many of us who work in an office setting, getting time outside and on grass can be difficult to squeeze into your day. I make it a point to go for a walk outside during my lunch breaks every day. I'll find an isolated spot, lie down on the grass, and unbutton my shirt for maximum vitamin D absorption (I make sure I'm far away from anyone first!). To be fair, I have a quiet park next to my work building, and I understand not everyone has access to green spaces near their work. But if you can, try to get sun exposure every day.

Intermittent Fasting

Intermittent fasting (IF) is an eating protocol of caloric restriction during certain hours of the day. The idea is the longer you aren't eating, the more time you're giving your body a chance to rest from digestion and allow the natural healing processes to take place. Prolonged fasts are not recommended for people who have recently been sick or are struggling with severe symptoms. If you've just been infected or are struggling with severe symptoms, I recommend loading up on fruits and vegetables regularly to give your body a continuous supply of the vitamins and minerals it needs to fight off the infection and heal.

Why is this important for people suffering from Long Covid? Several studies have found people with the disease have significantly higher levels of fasting glucose and insulin levels in their blood than healthy people. Due to the chronic infection, the body is in a highly inflamed and stressed state for a much longer period than normal. The elevated stress causes the body to convert its own muscle and organ proteins into glucose for energy. If this continues, the body can develop insulin resistance without the person consuming any processed sugary food.

The most popular method of IF is the 16:8 eating window, where you fast for 16 hours and eat within an 8-hour period. Typically, this is done by having your last meal of the day at 6 pm and holding off on eating until 10 am the following day. You can of course, change the hours around to what suits you, but most people find this to be the accessible form of IF.

The explanation for why the human body releases growth hormones when fasting goes back to the early days of our evolution. Humans didn't evolve to always have food on hand. We had to wake up and go hunt for our next meal, which could take up to several days. To keep our bodies strong, growth hormone keeps our muscles maintained and a process called autophagy begins.

Autophagy is a natural cellular process that involves the breakdown and recycling of damaged and dysfunctional cellular components. It clears out damaged proteins, decreases the risk of developing degenerative diseases such as cancer and Alzheimer's.

In this fasted state, the body switches from running on glycogen (sugar) to ketones (fat). Ketones are a much cleaner source of energy for the body and naturally produce no inflammation when being used. The low levels of inflammation also contribute to a very clear mental state, kind of like the background noise in your head becoming much quieter.

Intermittent fasting helped me recover. I've never been much of a morning person, so putting off breakfast for a few hours to catch up on the news or household chores works well for me. I don't recommend fasting if you have a stressful job or like to train in the morning. Some people prefer it, but I've always found I need to have something solid in my stomach before I can turn on my "turbocharger" for the day. On the weekends, or when I'm on holiday, I'll put off my first meal until about 10 am depending on when I had dinner. It gives me a chance to wake up and consider my plans for the day with absolute clarity.

Earlier in the book, I mentioned that vitamin C and glucose have a similar molecular structure and compete for absorption in the body. This is why eating foods low in carbohydrates and high in vitamin C in the morning is so beneficial. With your body running on ketones, there is no competition for vitamin C to be absorbed, and it can be utilized at maximum uptake efficiency.

I don't recommend prolonged fasts for someone in the acute phase of infection or struggling with severe symptoms. The body is craving nutrients to support the immune system and antioxidants to lower inflammation. Holding off on breakfast till a little later in the morning is fine, but anything longer will put yourself at risk of a nutrient deficiency.

Besides all the wonderful benefits of fasting mentioned above, the most important thing it does for us is improve our insulin response. Insulin is a hormone that is produced by the pancreas to reduce levels of sugar in our blood. It transports the "blood sugar" into our cells for energy. Think of insulin as the key that unlocks the door to a cell to let energy in. In a healthy person, who eats natural whole foods, their body doesn't need much insulin to add energy to its cells. However, for people who consume sugary processed carbohydrate-rich foods, their bodies need much higher amounts of insulin to keep this process going.

If they continue to abuse sugar and processed carbohydrates, a condition arises where the cells become less responsive to the effects of insulin, known as insulin resistance. Slowly, the pancreas compensates for this by producing more insulin to lower blood sugar. This can lead to a viscous cycle, where the body is producing more insulin to transport energy into the cells, but the cells are becoming more resistant to the effects of insulin.

This can happen to some degree for a person suffering from Long Covid/CFS, even without consuming large quantities of sugary foods. The elevated stressed state the viral infection puts you in causes your body to break down its own tissues for glucose. With enough time, this can also spiral to insulin resistance.

The insulin resistant state has many levels to it. The longer it goes untreated, the harder it becomes to recover from. Eventually, it can progress to type 2 diabetes, where a person has chronically high levels of blood sugar, but exceptionally low energy because insulin can't do its job. Even with insulin injections, the cells refuse to allow glucose inside.

The best way to avoid this is to practice intermittent fasting and rarely consume processed carbohydrates (especially sugars), avoid chronic stress from life and viral infections.

Long Covid and CFS are complicated multi-faceted issues. There is unfortunately, no one silver bullet that can take you back to health. Intermittent fasting is a tool you can use to treat yet another problem the disease causes in the body.

If you'd like to learn more about insulin resistance and how foods affect it, Dr Eric Berg has made countless videos on YouTube explaining just about everything there is about the subject.

Another expert I recommend is Jessie Inchauspe. She has written two books on how to manage your glucose levels and optimize the insulin response. Jessie went through a difficult health crisis several years ago and was forced to learn everything she could to get back to living a normal life.

A Summary of the Key Benefits of Fasting:

- Increases Growth Hormone (repairs cells, skin, muscles, lowers fat)
- Autophagy clears out dead cells and cancerous cells
- Boosts the immune system
- Stabilises blood sugar and drops Insulin down to zero
- Improves cognition
- Lowers inflammation in the body

When coming back to exercise, start SLOW and GENTLY

When I started to recover and regain some confidence, I quickly threw myself back into high-intensity training and weightlifting. Surely, after several months, I was in the clear, right? While the acute infection may have passed, the battle still waged on in the background. I soon found myself crashing from PEM for days afterwards.

Your body needs ample time to heal from the damage the virus and the inflammation has done to you. If you push too hard too early, you can reactivate the virus and set yourself back weeks.

For a healthy person, adopting the attitude of no pain, no gain does generally yield great results. This mindset allows you to push past your limits and grow. However, while recovering from a persistent virus, you need to reframe how you approach exercise. You must do less than what you previously were capable of and slowly increase the load you put onto your body. Until you become aware of your new limits, working out at a moderate to high intensity is too much of a risk to your recovery.

For someone who truly enjoys pushing past the limit, this is heartbreaking news. I've always felt so good when I've smashed a previous personal best in the gym or climbed an even bigger hill than I thought I was capable of on my bike. For some time, you will need to let go of these types of ambitions and focus on your recovery.

To replace your previous exercise activities when you start to feel up for it, I recommend the following:

- Walking - Outside and being surrounded by nature during the day is best. Being around nature naturally calms us down and boosts our mental health. Getting sunshine also boosts the immune system and our well-being.

- E-bike cycling – Cycling on a regular pedal bike is often too difficult when recovering, especially if you live in a hilly area. Using an E-bike, the electric motor greatly assists your pedaling to the point where you are hardly exerting yourself at all. It's great low intensity exercise, and you can gradually increase your exertion based on how you're recovering. Plus, there are the mental health benefits of being outside in nature and getting sun exposure.

- Yoga - Not my favourite, but I do see the benefits. The gentle movements and deep breathing are amazing for your circulation. Moving our bodies in ways which are different from our normal routine activates muscles that don't get used regularly.
- Swimming - As long as it's easy casual swimming. Going out for an easy swim in the sun does wonders for your circulation and hormones. Because it's a low-impact activity, you can start at any capability level and slowly progress.
- Light weight-training - The idea is to use a weight you can do for very high reps. The goal is not to build muscle but to exercise and promote blood circulation around your body.

When you do feel like you are ready to start pushing yourself a little, ALWAYS warm up slowly. This allows you to feel out your body on the day and prevents any kind of lymphatic flow disruption from a sudden jolt of activity. A slow, gentle warm-up shouldn't just be for those recovering from a persistent virus; it prevents injuries by priming the body through optimal blood circulation and hormonal changes.

Most of us walk around life in our heads, worried about day-to-day chores or the latest drama on social media. The focus of energy is in our minds, and our bodies are left neglected. A slow warm-up gradually shifts the energy away from the mind and into our body. Pumping blood and nutrients to muscles and tissue that haven't been flushed out recently.

HOLISTIC HEALING

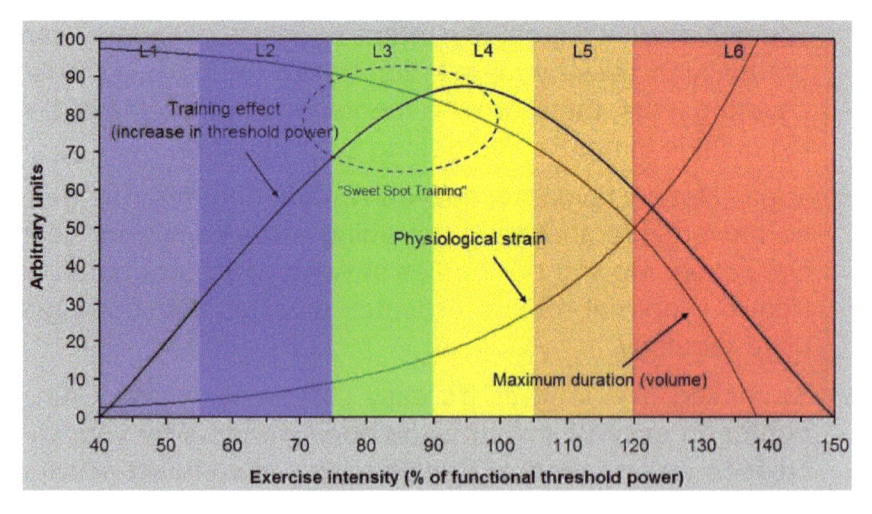

A critical component of returning to exercise or any activity is only operating within the "sweet spot" of exertion. You may have heard of the goldilocks story, where the young girl preferred the porridge that is neither too hot nor too cold but just the right temperature. This principle will apply to how you approach exercise; see the graph below.

You want to be staying in the green zone of activity. Too little and you will be bored; too much and you will crash. The trouble with recommending a range of exercise intensity or duration is that everyone will have different capabilities. A heart rate monitor can help with this if you are unsure of what the zones will feel like. However, we will discuss how to be mindful of your limits in the next section.

Listen to your body

Becoming mindful of your recovery ceiling will accelerate your recovery back to health. Knowing when your body can do more and when to take it easy is not a skill that's mastered overnight. This will be even more challenging now that your limits have drastically changed and how they can fluctuate from day to day. The frustrating part is the non-linear nature of the recovery. For example, going through a stressful period, such as an exam block or long days at work, will lower your capacity for exertion for a longer period of time than before. Being mindful of this reality will help you navigate your daily activities and regulate your mental health, as it can be easy to slip into negative self-talk while recovering.

With time, you'll begin to recognize the patterns and see the clues your body is trying to tell you. Some days, it won't be a good idea to push yourself. But on others, it will feel like you can do more. You'll develop a strong intuition into your own physiology, where you can pick up on the signals your body is putting out and interpret them accurately.

The first things I think about when I'm feeling run down are, am I getting enough vitamin C, vitamin D, and zinc. While I mentioned earlier it's important to plug all nutritional gaps; these three are the most important when it comes to energy and immune health. Keeping that first mental checklist small allows you to minimise the time you're thinking about your health and focus on your day. If problems persist, that's when you need to start going through what you've been eating and try to identify any further needs.

Sometimes, even if your nutrition and routine are on point, we just get tired. This is normal, even for healthy people. What's important is recognizing this and taking appropriate breaks. After my university exams, I rarely had enough money to travel abroad. I would book "staycations" in my home city for a few days to get away from my usual surroundings and unwind. Sure, I wasn't going anywhere new, but the change in scenery and routine was all I needed to reset my brain. Plus, there wasn't the trouble of dealing with airports or painfully long road trips to a destination.

The point is, what worked previously may not continue to work for you while you're recovering. Listening to your body and acting accordingly will help you come up with novel ways to maintain a healthy state of mind as you adapt to your recovery.

Get 7-9 Hours of quality sleep every night

Everyone knows you need to get decent sleep to operate at your best. We've all had late nights or cut sleep short, only to battle through fatigue, low energy, and brain fog for the following day. It isn't just your energy and focus that's affected by little sleep. Your immune system and hormones are also negatively impacted and will run in a sub-optimal state until a good night of sleep occurs. While the quantity of your sleep is crucial, the quality of your sleep can drastically improve your energy, focus, immune system, and your hormonal profile. Let's look at ways to increase the quality of sleep first, as generally if you are having quality sleep, it is easier to stay asleep.

To improve the quality of sleep:

1. Make your room as dark as possible
   - This doesn't mean just closing the curtains and doors. This means totally blocking out all possible light bleeding into your room. Under the doors, light seeping in through the blinds or thinly veiled curtains. The absolute worst is blue light from screens. These trick your brain into thinking it's daytime. So, a TV, monitor, or phone running while sleeping will hamper the quality of sleep immensely.
   - **Black-out curtains** are best to reduce light seepage. The budget alternative is buying large black garbage bags and taping them to your bedroom windows from the inside.
   - It can be a hassle getting to the light bleed from under doors. You can place towels at the base of your doors, but for the neat freaks like me out there, this gets frustrating every day. My alternative is getting a **sleep mask**. They are cheap, very easy to find online, and last forever if you treat them right.

2. Make your room as quiet as possible
   - Easy for some people, difficult for others. If you live in a rural area, it's probably easy to block out noise from your bedroom. All it can take is closing the windows and doors (while leaving a window slightly cracked open for fresh air). However, if you live in a dense urban setting, the background noise from traffic, other people, and building equipment can be hard to avoid.
   - The simplest way to block out sound is by using ear plugs or earmuffs while you sleep. Personally, I find ear plugs too intrusive to relax, but earmuffs can be purchased that are soft and squishy, so they won't press too hard on your ears or fall off during sleep.
   - It might be too much to ask to move to another area just for a quiet night's sleep, but if you are in the process of relocating, consider living on a quiet street and in a house where the rooms aren't exposed to the road.
3. No electronics/WIFI/phone signals

For many years, I thought there was no way these could affect someone's sleep and were just mumbo jumbo talking points from hypochondriacs. As I've gotten older and begun taking more on in life, I've noticed it can take much longer for me to get going in the morning. At first, I tried convincing myself it was just part of getting old, but it turns out that those people worried about electronics in the bedroom were really onto something.

For one week, I decided to leave my phone and laptop outside of my room while sleeping. While hard to gauge any tangible benefits immediately, I did feel more alert and was quicker to rise during that week. Thinking it could be down to other factors, I brought my phone and laptop to bed with me for a night and immediately noticed my sleep was poorer.

Any kind of electromagnetic field (EMF) produced from a device or power cable can have a negative effect on us. It may be impossible to avoid EMF's during the day in modern life, but limiting EMF exposure during sleep leads to better recovery both physically and mentally. This goes for WIFI signals too, as the EMF produced disrupts our ability to get into a deep sleep. To reduce EMF exposure during sleep, the steps below can help:

- No devices of any kind in your room, including any small wireless sensors that may be on the ceiling (I'll let you figure that out and decide if it is right for you)
- No wires or cables in the wall behind where you sleep.
- If you want A/C in your room, have it as far away from your bed as possible
- Avoid living next to powerlines, especially the big ones
- Use a Power switch timer for your WIFI router, so it turns off when you sleep, and back on in the morning automatically (see below)

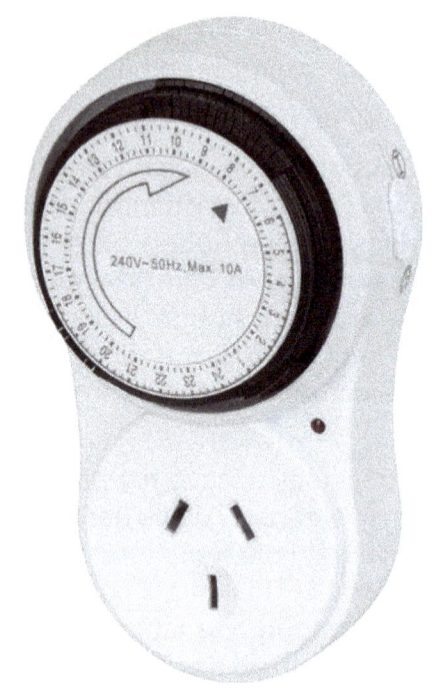

4. Keep Room temperature between 20-25 degrees Celsius or 68-77 degrees Fahrenheit

Depending on where you live, this can be difficult and expensive. I've lived in the north of Australia for most of my life, and air conditioner units are necessary to achieve these temperatures. Excessive heat and humidity will make it harder to fall and stay asleep. The trouble with the heat is there are only so many clothes you can take off to get comfortable. It can be inescapable, so sealing yourself off from the outside and blasting the A/C is the only real option.

The other end of the spectrum is excessive cold. Some people can tolerate colder temperatures better than others and don't mind putting on multiple layers of clothes. If temperatures drop below 18 degrees Celsius or 64 degrees Fahrenheit, it generally becomes harder to fall asleep if you're not prepared. Fortunately, modern A/C units are reverse systems that do both heating and cooling.

5. No drinking and eating within 1-2 hours of your bedtime

Doing either will make it harder to fall asleep and encourage waking up for the bathroom at night. Eating food turns your digestive system on and sends feel good neurotransmitters to the brain. Drinking will, at best, wake you up during the night to relieve yourself and at worst, prevent you from sleeping at all. It should be common sense, but any kind of caffeinated or sugary beverage consumed at night will make it harder to fall asleep and reduce the quality of said sleep.

- Don't eat a large meal or drink anything within 1-2 hours of your bedtime
- Leave at least 6 hours before bedtime if you are consuming caffeine (Cola's have caffeine too, albeit in smaller doses than coffee or energy drinks)

To Improve the Quantity of Sleep:

1. Following the quality of sleep measures will help you get more sleep. Generally, if you can achieve a deeper sleep state, it will be easier to stay asleep.
2. It's obvious, but being responsible with your sleep schedule by sleeping earlier and waking up later is the first place to start
3. Falling asleep isn't always easy, especially for anyone like me with an active mind. If you find yourself tossing and turning it could be caused by several things, but the primary reasons are stress being too high and/or a nutritional deficiency.

This can be like a negative feedback loop, with high levels of chronic stress taking up your nutritional resources to function and perform, and your immune system also demanding nutritional resources to deactivate the virus. When the body has no further resources for the immune system, the virus can reassert itself, Inflaming the body further and raising stress levels higher, making it harder to go to sleep.

- Too much stress (Remedy - go for a walk, read a book, watch a comfort TV show or journal what's going on inside your head)
- Nutritional deficiency - identify what kind of gap there could be from what you've eaten recently. Your immune system could be trying to get to work, but it doesn't have the tools it needs to get going. It's tricky to recommend foods or supplements that can help the immune system but also relax the mind. For me, avocados, potatoes, wild blueberries help extinguish any kind of immune flare-up and put my mind at ease. Marine Sourced Calcium supplements also work wonders in relaxing my muscles and mind, while giving me a great night's sleep.
- Another great tonic for sleep is the amino acid Glycine. Either in powder or pill form will work the same; it's best taken just before sleep to avoid any kind of drowsiness during the day. Research has found Glycine has a calming effect

on the brain and nervous system, reducing neuronal activity, anxiety and regulating body temperature. I always find I fall asleep faster and stay asleep much better when I take Glycine. The dreams are also particularly vivid too.

- Generally, Magnesium Glycinate is effective at relaxing the body too. There are many different types of Magnesium; each have a different effect on the body. Magnesium Glycinate has been found to be the most relaxing for both the body and mind. Perfect for sleep.

CHAPTER SUMMARY: WHAT TO START DOING

1. Supporting the Mitochondria
   - The cornerstone of recovering and getting your energy back
   - All roads lead back to dysfunctional mitochondria
2. Cover all of your nutritional bases by seeing what's in your food at www.cronometer.com
   - Every vitamin and mineral is important for your recovery
3. Having a natural vitamin C source in every meal
   - Vitamin C is water-soluble; you need it every 4 hours to prevent deficiencies while sick
   - Capsicum (red peppers), fruits, leafy greens, tomatoes, citrus fruits, and big salads are optimal
   - Extra Virgin Olive Oil aids in the absorption of vitamin C; apply it as a salad dressing
4. Use extra virgin olive oil everywhere
   - Significant part of why the Mediterranean diet is so healthy
   - Use it for cooking, salad dressing, dipping and marinades
5. Getting adequate Zinc from natural sources every day
   - Red meat, seafood, chicken
   - Limit foods with phytic acid (whole grains, nuts, seeds and legumes)

6. Consume as many vegetables as possible
   - Nearly all vegetables are packed with nutrients
7. Find a Greens powder that works for you
   - The best choices have spirulina and wheatgrass in them
8. When recovering, only eat chicken, lean beef, and wild-caught fish
   - Anything else can overload your lymphatic system and create a histamine response (inflammation)
9. Get at least 15 minutes of good sun exposure every day
   - The best time is sunrise and during the middle of the day
10. Try and implement intermittent fasting into your routine
    - It's great for the immune system, resets your hormones, and lowers inflammation
    - Having a late breakfast works for me and most people, but see what you like best.
11. When exercising, start SLOW and gently
    - Test the waters of your activity limits
    - Never exceed your capacity, stay in the "sweet spot" of exertion
12. Listen to your body
    - It gives you clues to the state of your body and what you are capable of
13. Get 7-9 hours of sleep every night
    - A non-negotiable for a strong immune system and swift recovery

CHAPTER 4

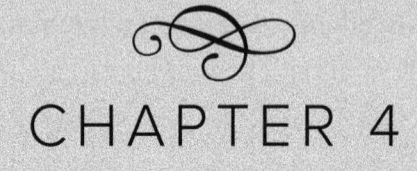

HEALING FOOD RECIPES

From all the books and recipes I've found for fighting off persistent viruses, many of the prescribed meals haven't been satisfying or lack the sufficient macronutrients I need to function. My approach to meal preparation covers all the essential vitamins and minerals, takes the least amount of time to prepare, is guaranteed to fill you up, and always tastes delicious.

Please note these meals may not be suitable for people with severe gut dysbiosis. If you're struggling with damage to your gut lining, you will need to focus on consuming foods and supplements that help restore your normal gut function. That's not to say the meals below will harm your gut lining; they just won't be the best starting place.

If you have the time to do a week of juice/fruit/vegetable fasts, then I recommend doing so. A diet of primarily vegetables and fruits will be great for making your blood more alkaline and delivering important nutrients around your body. You may also be suffering from severe symptoms that prevent you from consuming anything heavy, so for the time being, stick with fruits, vegetables, and maybe some lean meats.

When I went through my acute infection, I limited the amount of meat and heavy starches I was consuming. With enough time and patience, I slowly grew stronger and felt the need for more solid food in my stomach. This also was a sign that I could begin doing light exercises again. Below are my favourite recipes for healing and functioning at a high level.

BREAKFAST

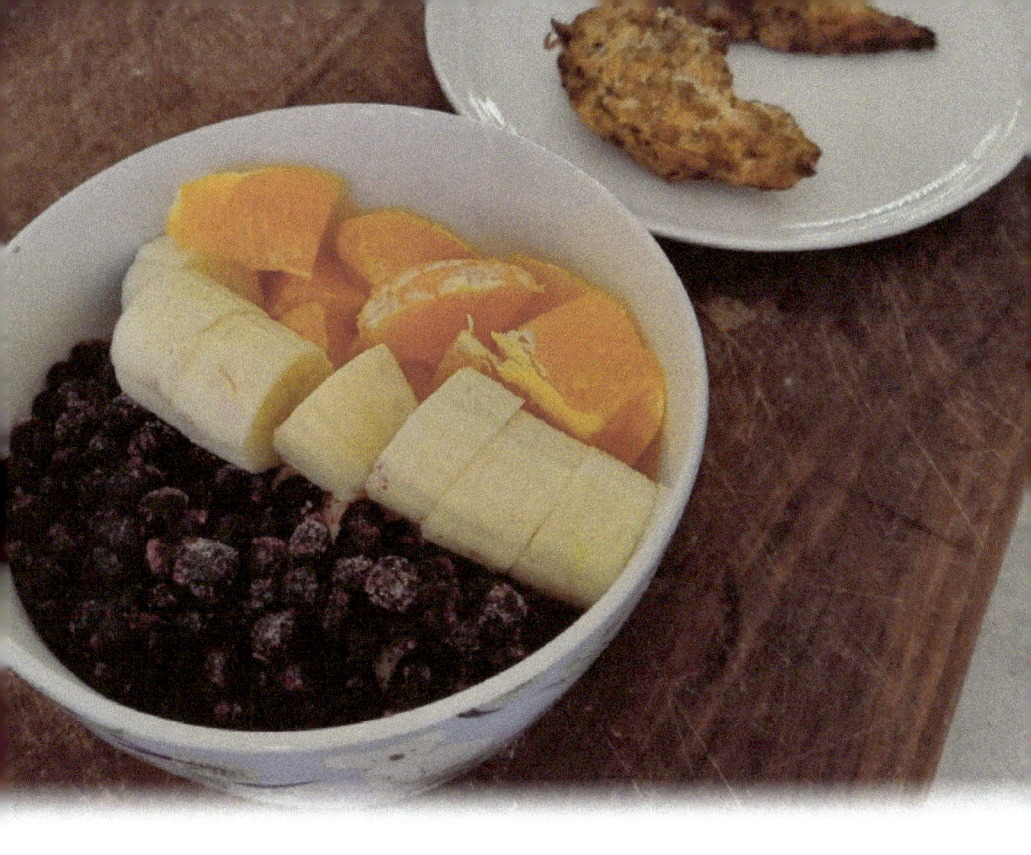

Fruit Salad w/ Chicken Breast/Nuts

Ingredients

- 1 Orange
- 1 Banana
- 50-100g of Wild Blueberries
- 100g Chicken Breast/ 50g Nuts

Super easy to make and tastes delicious. Chop up the banana and orange into a bowl and pour over the wild blueberries. They all mix together to create something better than the sum of their parts!

   As for the protein source, you can cook up some chicken breast with a seasoning to your liking and eat this as a side dish. Or grab a handful of almonds or cashew nuts. Your choice will come down to what your goals/lifestyle choices are. The chicken breast will provide more protein and has a different nutrient profile, making it better for more active people. Whereas nuts are super easy and nutrient dense, though they are lacking in protein compared to chicken.

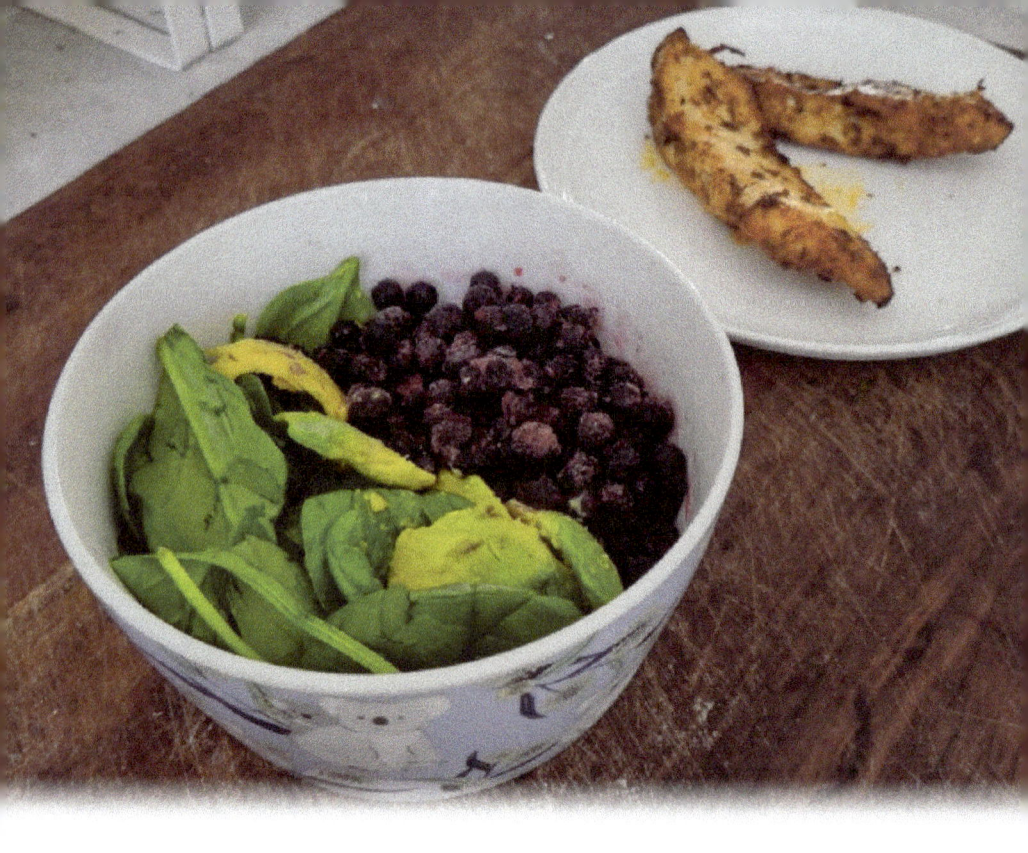

Spinach, Avocado, and Blueberry Salad w/ Chicken or Nuts

Ingredients

- 20-40g Spinach (1-2 handfuls)
- 50g Avocado
- 50-100g Wild Blueberries
- 100g Chicken breast/ 50g Nuts

This one is pretty out there, but I promise you it's a game-changer in the morning. A great alternative to fruit salad if you are concerned about weight loss or have a blood sugar problem. Wild blueberries are one of the lowest GI fruits in the world, have a powerful nutrient profile, and taste superb! They are different from regular cultivated blueberries, as they contain more skin than fruit (there are more nutrients in the skin), have less sugar, and far more antioxidants. Your normal supermarket isn't likely to have them, so you may need to track them down from a health food store. I promise you they'll be worth it.

If you can't get your hands on wild blueberries, then cultivated berries still provide numerous health benefits and taste great.

Grab a handful of spinach, avocado, and wild blueberries throw them all in a decently tall bowl, and mix them up. The creamy avocado mixes with the sweet blueberries and spinach to make a surprisingly tasty green salad for breakfast. For the protein source, use chicken breast or a high-protein nut.

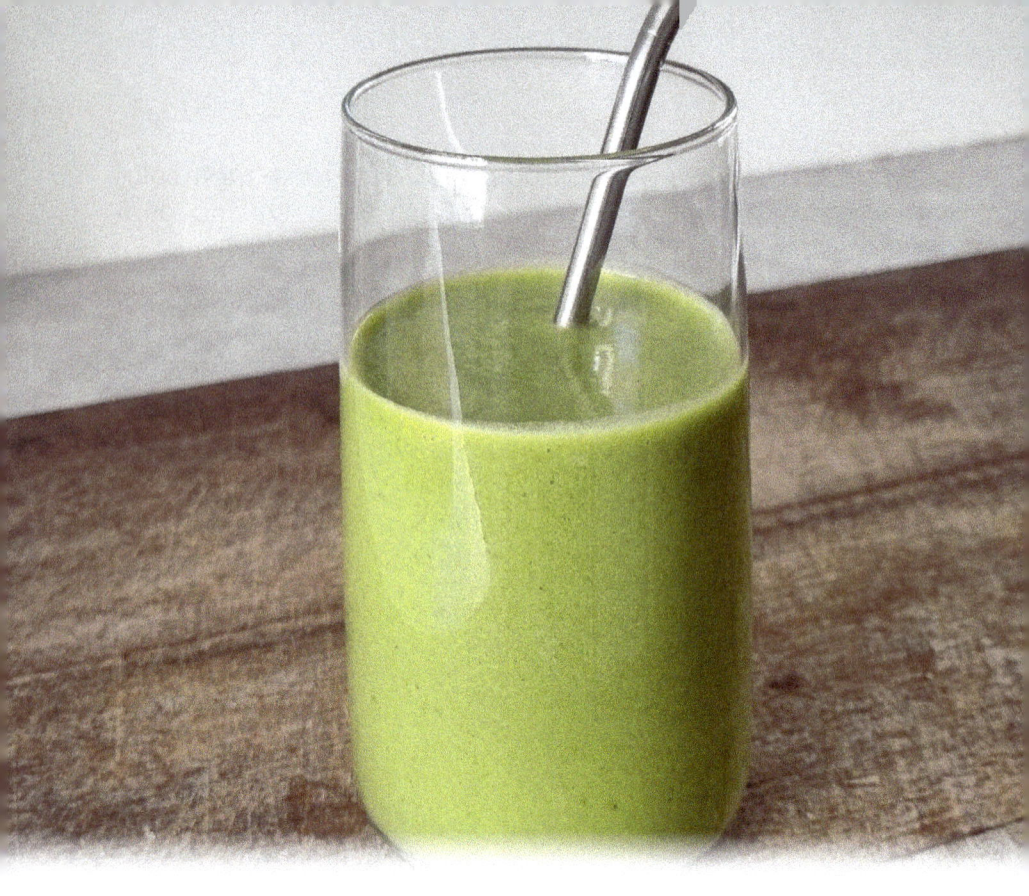

Breakfast Smoothie

- 20-40g Spinach
- 25g Avocado
- 1 Banana
- 1 Tablespoon Natural Peanut Butter
- 1 Scoop of Chocolate Vegan Protein Powder

Immune Boosting, cleansing, and alkalizing, this smoothie is loaded with energy and protein. The taste is superb and goes down quickly. If you need a clean energy boost for a workout in the morning, give this a try. It's easy to make and bolsters your immune system, replenishing and priming your adrenal glands for a solid workout. I throw everything into a "Bullet" style blender with about 300-400 ml of water and wizz it all up. You can also use any kind of nut milk, though I'd steer clear of any soy-based products or any with added sugar.

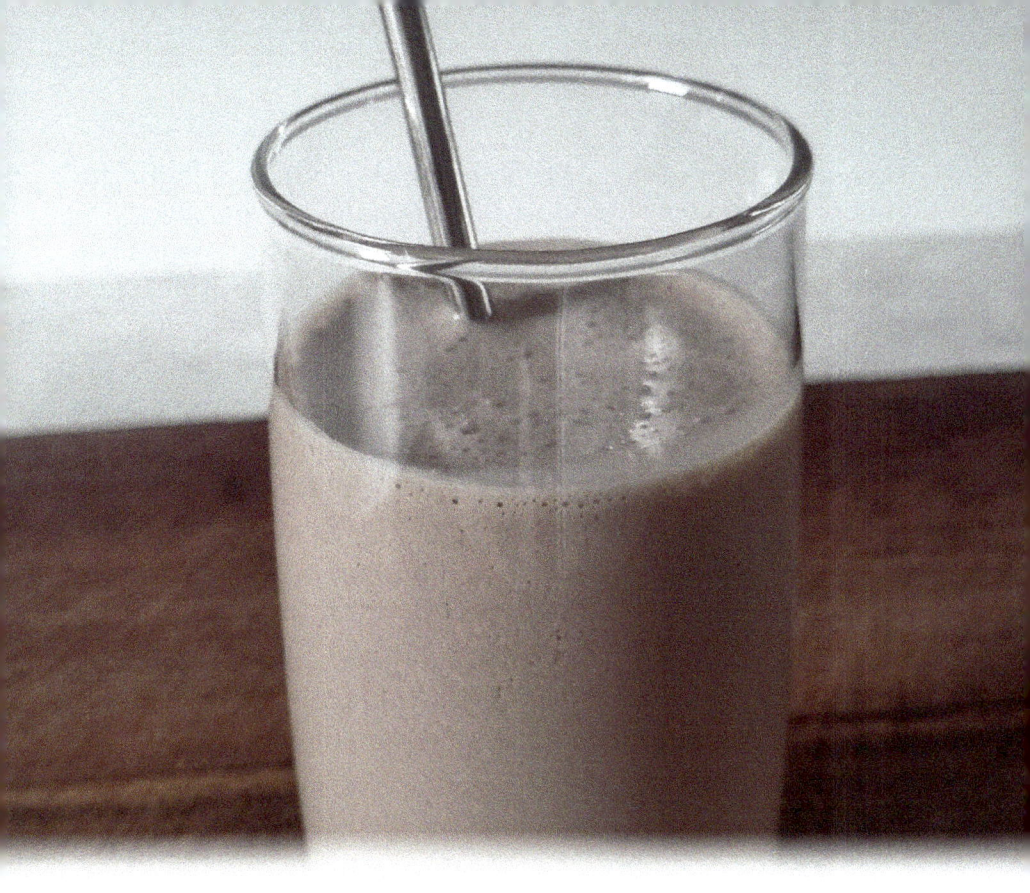

Anti-Inflammatory Gut Healing Smoothie

- 20g Turmeric
- 20g Ginger
- 1 Teaspoon Raw Cacao Powder
- 1 Teaspoon Raw Unheated Honey
- 300-400ml Organic Kefir
- Sprinkle of Black Pepper (Piperine)

A powerhouse for lowering inflammation all over your body, rebuilding your gut microbiome, and healing your damaged vasculature. This smoothie surprisingly has a "cola" like taste to it, providing you get premium kefir. Wonderful for the immune system, this smoothie will lower inflammation all over your body and allow it to kickstart the healing process.

Like all smoothies, it's easy to make. Simply peel the ginger and turmeric and chop into small chunks; add to your blender with everything else, and spin it all up. The black pepper has something in it called piperine, which activates the turmeric. The only milk product I recommend is organic kefir for the base. This covers up the strong ginger and turmeric taste. Some people do well with raw cow milk, but I always feel bloated and foggy after consuming it, so I steer clear.

Kefir is also amazing for rebuilding your gut. It's absolutely loaded with friendly bacteria, containing up to 50 billion live active species and over 20 billion colony-forming units (CFUs). Yogurt typically has 1-5 live species and 6 billion CFUs.

Ginger has several bioactive compounds that contribute to the immune system and health. Its primary compound, Gingerol, lowers inflammation and has a strong antioxidant effect.

Turmeric, like Ginger has highly nutritious, with the main compound in it being curcumin. Curcumin has been well-studied for its anti-inflammatory and antioxidant properties.

MAIN COURSES
(CAN BE LUNCH OR DINNER)

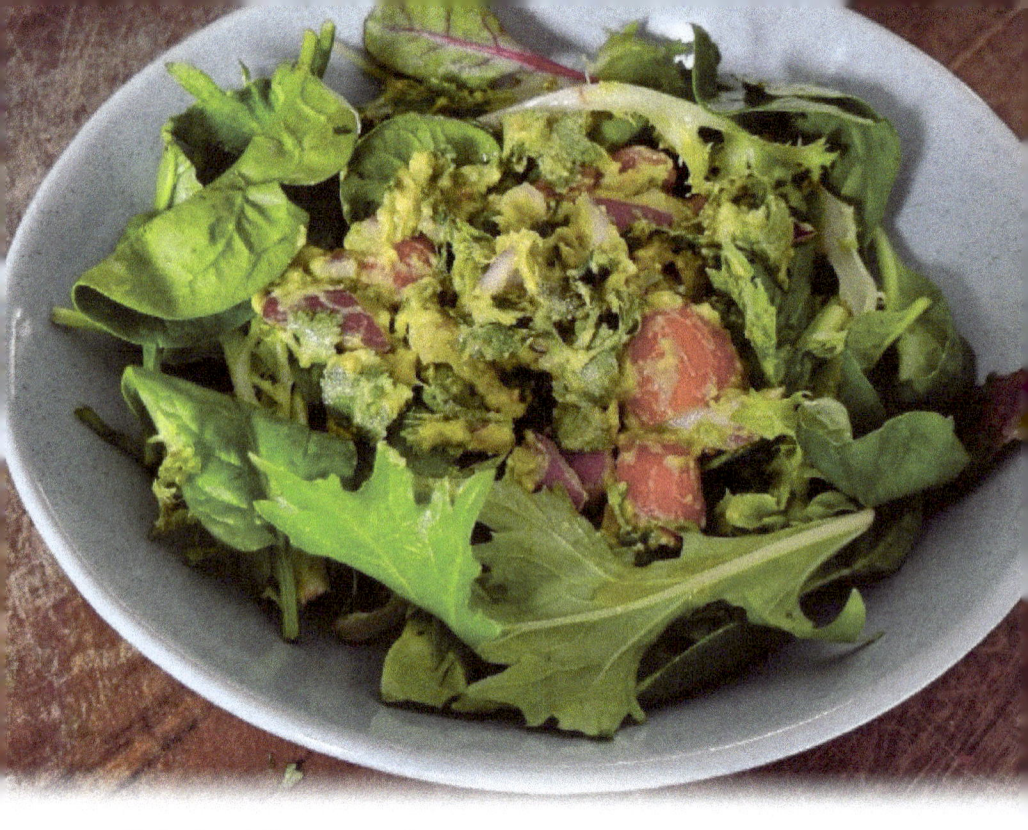

Salad w/ Guacamole

Ingredients

- Few handfuls of Mixed Salad leaf (Rocket, Spinach, Lettuce, etc)
- 50g Cucumber
- ½ Avocado
- 4 Cherry Tomatoes
- ¼ Red Onion
- Coriander
- ½ Lime Juiced
- 1 teaspoon Salt
- Few drops of Tabasco or Chili Sauce
- Drizzle of Extra Virgin Olive Oil (EVOO) as dressing

When I got serious about improving my diet, I decided I would try eating 7-10 cups of vegetables each day and see if it was worth the hype. Dr Berg recommended eating a big salad every day as the easiest way to get those numbers up.

Did it make a difference?

I would say this new habit has been the cornerstone of my recovery from both CFS and Long Covid. Nearly every day since 2018, I've had some kind of salad before my lunch, and it has drastically improved my recovery, energy, and clarity. When I go a day without a salad, I feel like there's something not quite right, and I've cheated myself.

Without a doubt, whenever I'm feeling a little drained or think a cold is coming on, I'll make extra sure to have a big salad that day to keep myself soldiering on.

Beside all the vitamins and minerals in green leafy vegetables, there are nitrates in them as well. Nitrates are a precursor to nitric oxide which supports your blood vessels and arteries to pump blood around your body.

You can add nearly any kind of vegetable to a salad. Peppers, snow peas, asparagus, or tomatoes. The trick to enjoying salads is adding EVOO, avocado, and a pinch of salt to bring it all together. Otherwise, munching into all those vegetables will make you feel like a rabbit. I prefer to put Guacamole on my salads, but when I'm pressed for time, EVOO, avocado, and salt work quite well.

1. Grab Salad leaves put into a big bowl, and drizzle over EVOO
2. Peel the cucumber and chop into chunks; place over the salad leaves
3. Make Guacamole and put on top Salad

Guacamole

1. Cut an avocado in half and extract one side of it into a tall bowl.
2. Squeeze half a lime's juice into the bowl, add the tabasco sauce and salt.
3. Get a fork and mush it all up together until it is fairly smooth and runny
4. Add chopped tomatoes, chopped onion, chopped coriander and mix it all up

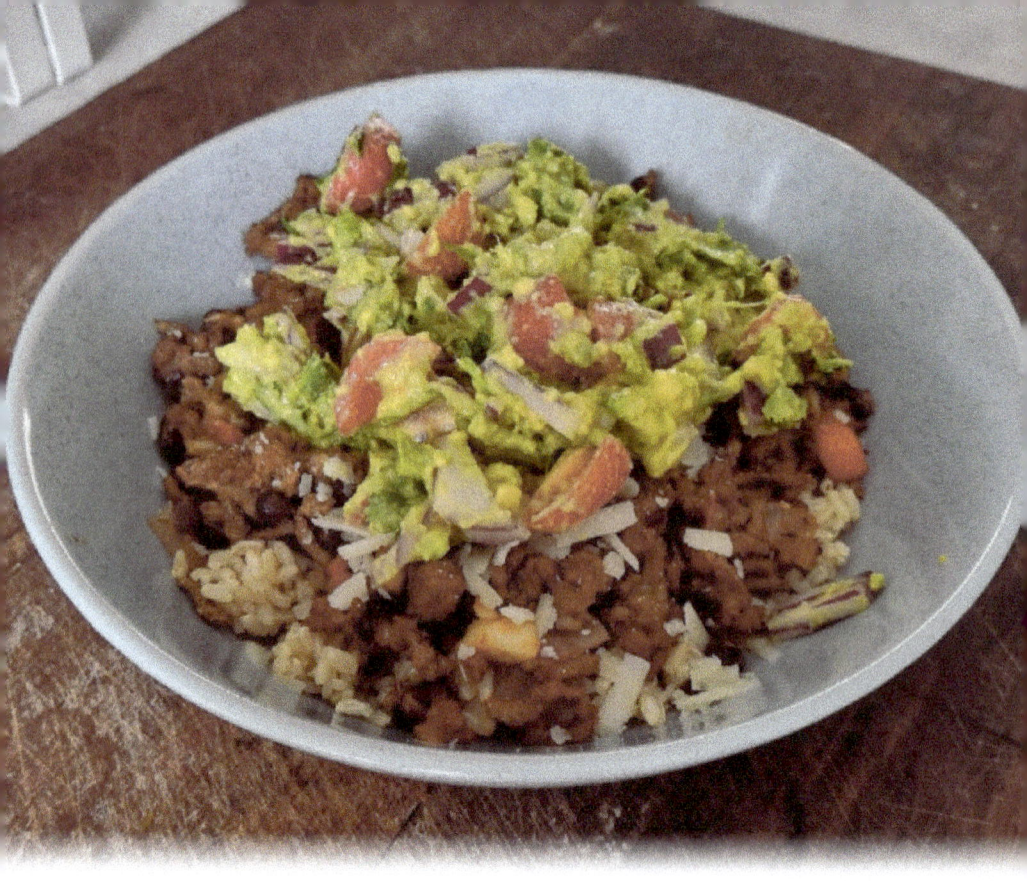

Mexican Chili Con Carne w/ Guacamole

Ingredients

- 500g Premium Beef Mince
- 1 entire bulb of Garlic
- 1 Red/Brown Onion
- ½ Red Capsicum
- 1 table spoon Extra Virgin Olive Oil
- 1-2 400g tins of Black/Pinto Beans
- 1 200g can Diced Tomatoes
- Mexican Spice Mix
- 1 tablespoon Smoked Paprika
- 1 tablespoon ground Cumin
- 1 teaspoon ground coriander

- ½ teaspoon ground chilli
- ½ teaspoon chilli flakes
- 1 teaspoon dried oregano flakes
- 1 teaspoon dried thyme
- 1 teaspoon salt
- 1 teaspoon black pepper
- 40ml water
- 280g Brown Rice cooked
- 30g Parmesan Cheese

Guacamole

- ½ an avocado
- ½ lime
- 50g of tomato (small tomatoes or 1 big one)
- Coriander
- ½ red onion
- ½ teaspoon salt
- Few drops of tabasco sauce or a pinch of chilli powder

This one is a heavy hitter. Loaded with high-quality macro and micronutrients, this meal is enormously satisfying, immune boosting and is sure to impress your friends. I developed this when I needed a cheap lunch that fortified my immune system but kept me full for hours and also giving me an "edge" in life.

1. First thing is to de-skin the garlic chop it up, and leave for at least 10 minutes. This is IMPORTANT; you must allow the garlic to be exposed to air to turn on and amplify the amazing benefits of allicin, the most bioactive compound in garlic. Allicin is a potent antiviral and antioxidant. It also is great for your vasculature.
2. Mix the paprika, cumin, ground coriander, ground chili, chili flakes, dried oregano, dried thyme, salt, black pepper, and water in a bowl until all clumped together.

3. Start cooking the rice in whichever way you prefer. I use a rice cooker because it's easy and idiot-proof.
4. Get a fry pan heated up to medium with extra virgin olive oil and cook the beef mince till it's all brown.
5. Add the chopped onions into the cooked beef and sauté for about 2 minutes
6. Add the chopped red capsicum and sauté for about 2 minutes
7. Add the chopped garlic and only cook for 1 minute to preserve its nutrients (IMPORTANT)
8. Add the Mexican spice mix and diced tomatoes, and get it all mixed up. If you use heaps of diced tomatoes, you'll need to let it simmer for a long time to reduce the water. If you only use a small can, 10 minutes is adequate.
9. Open up the can of beans and strain them out in a colander, wash off all the liquid they put in the can to preserve it. Add the washed beans to the chilli and stir them in.
10. The rice should be cooked by now. If not, let the chilli con carne simmer at a lower temperature and start on the guacamole!

Guacamole

1. Cut an avocado in half and extract one-half of the contents into a tall bowl.
2. Squeeze half a lime's juice into the bowl, add the tabasco sauce and salt.
3. Get a fork and mush it all up together until it is fairly smooth and runny
4. Add chopped tomatoes, chopped onion, chopped coriander and mix it all up

To serve, I add a layer of rice to the bottom of a bowl, followed by the chilli Mix and the guacamole on top. The Chilli con Carne is an absolute staple of mine. I've been making it every Saturday for years, and every time I make it, I fall in love all over again.

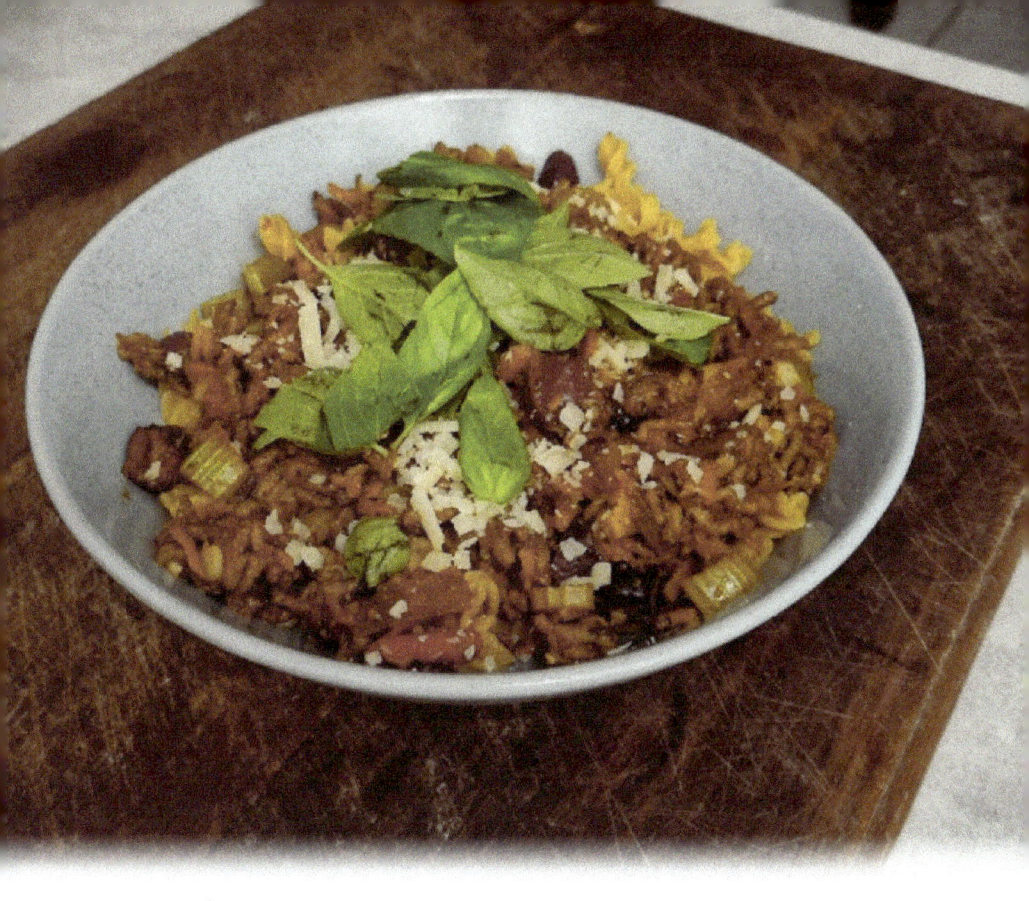

Spaghetti Bolognese

Ingredients

- 350g Lentil Pasta/Spaghetti
- 500g Premium Beef Mince
- 1 400g tin Diced Tomatoes
- 1 Carrot
- 1 Clove of garlic
- 1 Onion
- 50g Black Olives
- ½ teaspoon of Chilli flakes
- ½ teaspoon of Salt
- ½ teaspoon of Black Pepper
- 1 teaspoon of Thyme

- 1 teaspoon of Oregano
- 1 teaspoon of Basil seasoning
- 1 handful of Fresh Basil Leaves
- ½ tablespoon of Extra Virgin Olive Oil

A staple meal for many households. Spaghetti Bolognese can be made in all sorts of variations. This iteration focuses on preserving nutrition while keeping it tasty and convenient.

1. Heat up a frying pan on medium heat with the extra virgin olive oil
2. Crush the garlic with a knife, peel the skins off, and let it sit for 10 minutes to activate the wonderful benefits of the allicin.
3. Chop up the onion, peel the carrot, and shred to your liking
4. Place the mince meat into the medium-heated frying pan and break apart with a spatula until all the mince is brown and cooked
5. Add the onions to the pan and stir them in for 2 minutes, then add the carrots and cook for another 2 minutes, followed by the garlic, cooking for 1 minute and stirring
6. Add the tin of diced tomatoes, chili flakes, salt, pepper, thyme, oregano, and basil, stirring everything together until it's an even consistency. Reduce the temperature to low and let simmer for about 10 minutes
7. Cook the spaghetti in boiling water until it is al dente (not too soft and not too hard)
8. Plate up with the spaghetti first, the Bolognese, parmesan cheese to your taste, and chopped fresh basil leaves. Drizzle over some EVOO for the authentic Italian touch

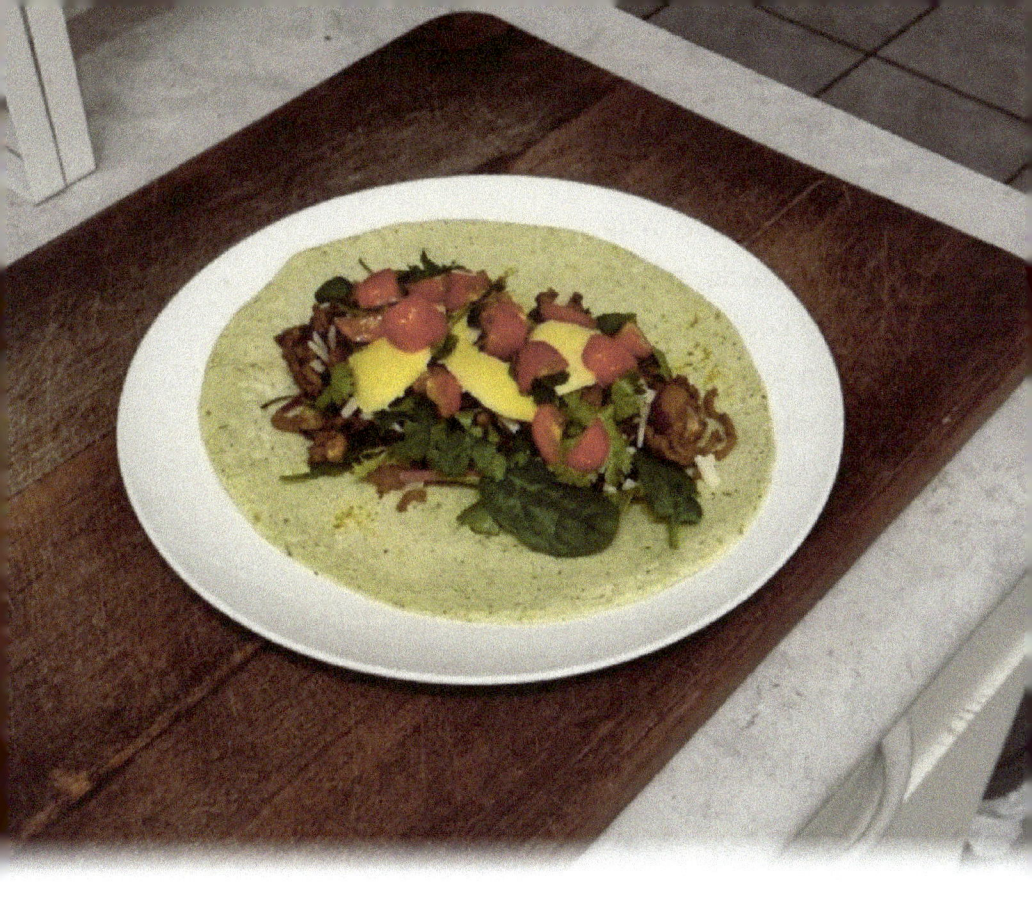

Mexican Chili Beef Wraps

- Ingredients
- 250-500g Premium Beef Mince (Depending on serving size)
- Spinach Wraps
- 1 Onion
- 1 clove of garlic
- 400g Can of Black Beans
- 100g of Red Capsicum
- 1 tsp of Cumin
- 1 tsp of Smoke Paprika
- ½ tsp of Thyme
- ½ tsp of Oregano
- ½ tsp of Salt (or to taste)

- ½ tsp of Black Pepper
- Chili Flakes to taste
- Chili Powder to taste
- 100g Leafy Salad mix
- ½ an Avocado
- 10 Baby Tomatoes
- 1 Pickled Jalapeno
- 25g Coriander/Cilantro
- 15g shredded Parmesan cheese

    Similar to the Chili con Carne w/ rice, follow the instructions to make the same beef mix but without the can of diced tomatoes. Put the chili mix into a wrap with the leafy salad mix, avocado, tomatoes, cheese, and coriander. It's easy to make, easy to clean up, tastes great, and most importantly, you get all the macro and micronutrients you need.

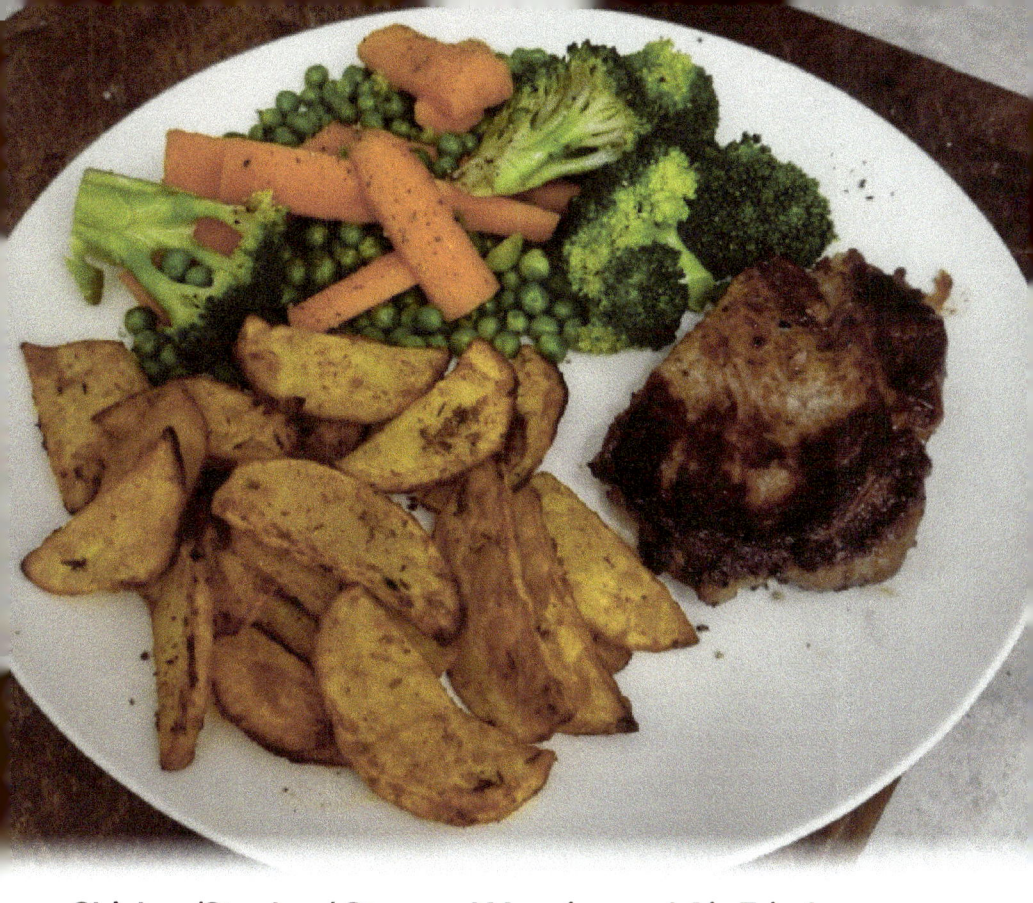

Chicken/Steak w/ Steamed Veggies and Air Fried Potatoes

Ingredients

- 150g of either Chicken Breast or Steak
- ¼ of a Broccoli head
- 1 cup of Peas
- 1 medium sized Carrot
- 3 medium sized potatoes
- 1 tbsp of Extra Virgin Olive Oil
- ½ tsp of Salt
- ½ tsp of Black Pepper
- ½ tsp of smoked paprika
- ½ tsp of Oregano
- ½ tsp of Thyme

Your classic meat, potatoes, and veggies main course. This is simple, easy to make, with the right spices delicious, and loaded with all the vitamins and minerals your body needs to recover.

1. Peel potatoes and slice into chip-size chunks however you like them. Put all sliced potatoes into a large bowl with extra virgin olive oil, oregano, smoked paprika, thyme, and salt, and give them a good mix around with your hands until all the potatoes are covered evenly.
2. Put seasoned potatoes into an Air Fryer for 12-15 minutes at 200 degrees C or in a conventional oven for 20 minutes at 200 degrees C.
3. While the potatoes are cooking, heat up a frying pan on medium to high heat. If using chicken, slice the breast in two to allow for faster cooking.
4. Season your chicken or steak with extra virgin olive oil, salt, and pepper until all sides are evenly covered.
5. Cook the steak for 5 minutes on each side, turn off the stove, turn the steak once more, and let rest on the cooling down fry pan for 5 minutes
6. For Chicken, cook for 3 minutes on one side, then flip and cook for 8 minutes, turn off the stove, flip chicken once more, and let rest for 5 minutes on the cooling fry pan
7. Chop up the broccoli into bite-sized florets, peel the carrots, and chop into quarters
8. Chop up the carrots in whichever way pleases you
9. Steam the vegetables in this order while keeping them all in the steamer, carrots first for 4 minutes, broccoli for 4 minutes, and finally, the peas for 3 minutes
10. Ready to plate up, put all the items onto a plate, and drizzle some extra virgin olive oil over the steamed vegetables and crack a little pepper over them, too for some extra flavour.

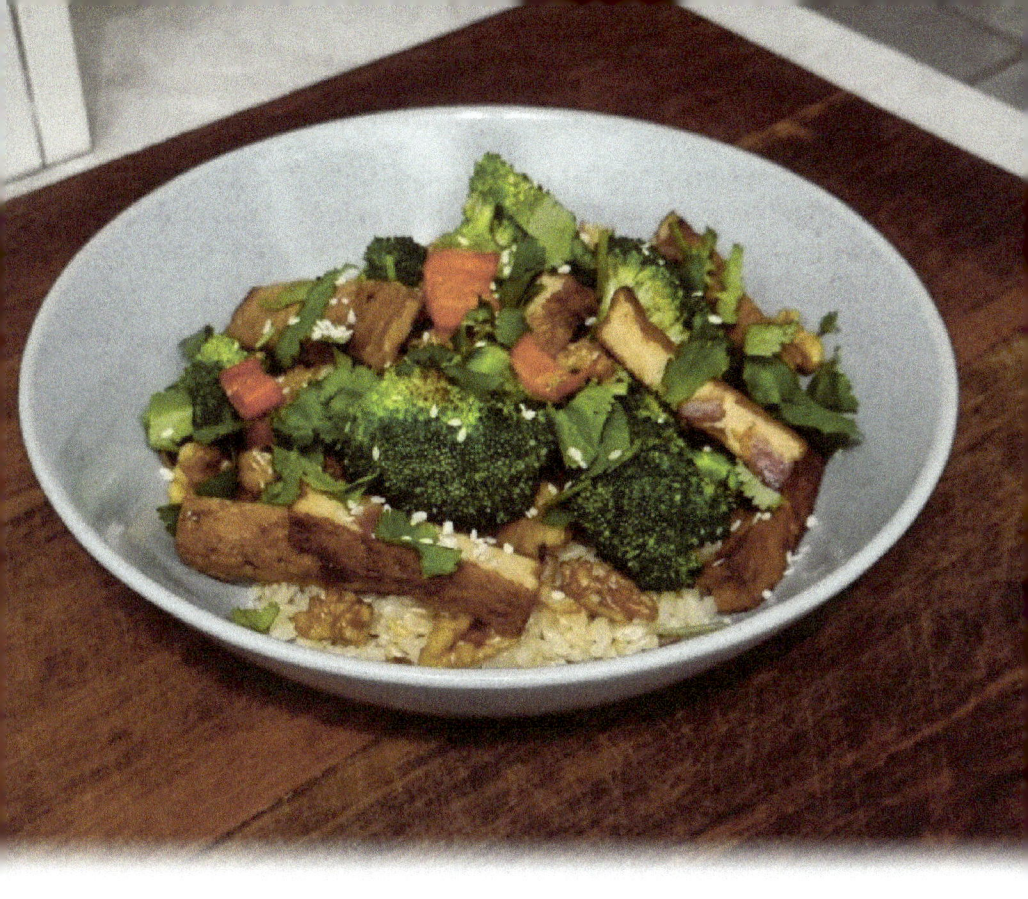

Tofu/Tempe Walnut & Veggie Stir fry w/ brown rice

Ingredients

- 400g of Tofu/Tempeh
- 60g Walnuts
- 1 head of Broccoli
- 1 medium size Chili
- 1 Onion
- 4 Cloves of Garlic
- 1 tsp honey
- 2 tsp Soy sauce
- 1 small bunch Coriander
- 2 cups Brown Rice
- 2 Tablespoons of water

A great vegan dish that is satisfying, tasty, and covers many nutritional bases. Like all my favourite recipes, it's simple to put together and easy to make. The tofu/tempeh are a good base, and the Walnuts add a crunch to the palette.

1. Mix the honey and soy sauce together until the honey has completely liquified.
2. Cook 2 cups of brown rice
3. Chop up the garlic, chilli, onion, broccoli
4. Heat a wok over high heat with extra virgin olive oil and stir fry the walnuts for 2 minutes until they are golden. Transfer to a bowl to cool down.
5. Using the same wok, stir-fry the onion for 2 minutes, add the garlic and chili stir-frying for another minute, add the broccoli and two tablespoons of water, stirring for two more minutes. The water will steam up and make the broccoli bright green and crispy.
6. Add the honey soy sauce mixture, walnuts, and tofu/tempeh into the wok and stir fry for 2 minutes
7. Plate up, dividing the brown rice and stir fry mixture. Garnish with coriander leaves over the dish

CHAPTER 5

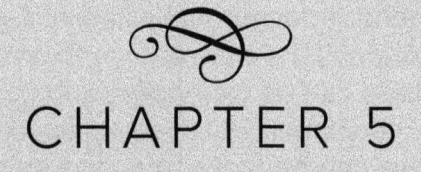

NUTRITIONAL SUPPLEMENTS

'd like to preface this section by saying it's always best to get vitamins and minerals from natural sources. Most vitamins and minerals in pill form are produced at very low standards, and either aren't absorbed well or not at all. They can come in many forms, such as magnesium chelate, zinc oxide, and calcium citrate. Some of these are better absorbed than others, but at the end of the day, natural sources will exceed these significantly.

I only recommend a decent multivitamin if you are pressed for time/money or don't have the energy to prepare good food. I get it; healthy food can be expensive, and cooking it yourself is a big energy consumer. But loading up on synthetic vitamins and minerals can be ineffective and detrimental to your health. Taking excessive vitamin C can interfere with copper absorption, and excessive zinc can hinder iron absorption. All vitamins and minerals are in a synergistic dance together, and both deficiencies and excesses can lead to problems.

For those struggling with severe long-haul symptoms and aren't physically capable of cooking healthy meals for themselves, I strongly urge you to reach out to anyone close to help you cook your meals. Supplementation should just be that, a supplement to your diet. It should never replace balanced, complete foods.

If you are serious about getting better, you'll need to put some effort into learning what foods to buy and how to prepare them. The previous chapter gives you some ideas on where to start. Your recovery time will dramatically decrease if you give your body high-quality nutrition. That being said, let's discuss some of the supplements that helped me the most.

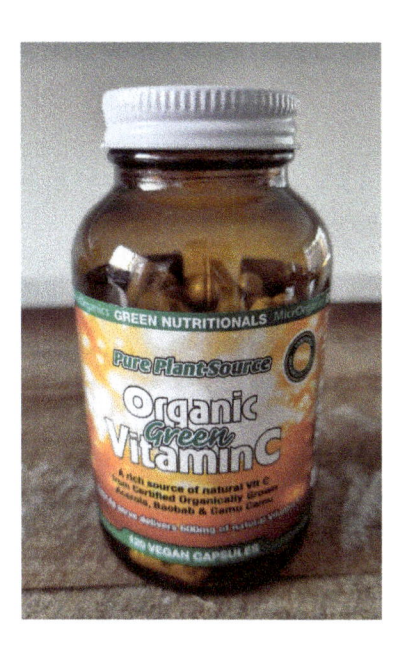

Natural Vitamin C

There are two kinds of Vitamin C, L-ascorbic acid and D-ascorbic acid.

L-ascorbic acid is Vitamin C in its **natural** form, found in citrus fruits and vegetables. D-ascorbic acid is **synthetically** produced from corn starch. It's broken down in a process that uses high heat, enzymes, and acetone to extract the ascorbic acid. All the phytonutrients found in natural Vitamin C are lost in this process, leaving a dead husk that offers little nutritional value.

In the early days of my infection, I bought a big bottle of 1000 chewable ascorbic acid vitamin C tablets. They tasted great, were cheap, and nearly every supermarket had some on the shelf. Even with me sucking down 10 of those a day, I barely noticed any kind of improvement in my recovery. It wasn't until a friend told me about natural Vitamin C supplements that I began doing further research.

Eventually, I came across a company with a great reputation that had a natural vitamin C product. Visiting my local health store, I bought a bottle downed a few capsules on the drive home without any water. Almost immediately, I felt my body relax and my symptoms dissipate, telling me this was the real deal.

In its natural state, vitamin C is a compound of several different elements and trace minerals, as well as ascorbic acid. Combined, they have a synergistic effect and equal more than the sum of their parts.

If you see a vitamin C tablet or capsule, chances are it's synthetic, only containing the ascorbic acid component. Meaning you miss out on the other parts of natural vitamin C. If you want to get the good stuff, it mostly comes from fruits with exceptionally high vitamin C content, such as camu camu, sea buckthorn, acerola, and baobab. If you can find a natural vitamin C product with all these plants in it, you can rest assured it's worth it.

Vitamin C is essential for numerous roles in the body. It is critical we get ample amounts everyday. Below are some of the other benefits it provides:

- A powerful antioxidant that reduces inflammation and prevents arterial plaquing
- Greatly improves iron absorption especially from plant sources
- A large component of collagen formation keeping skin firm and gums healthy

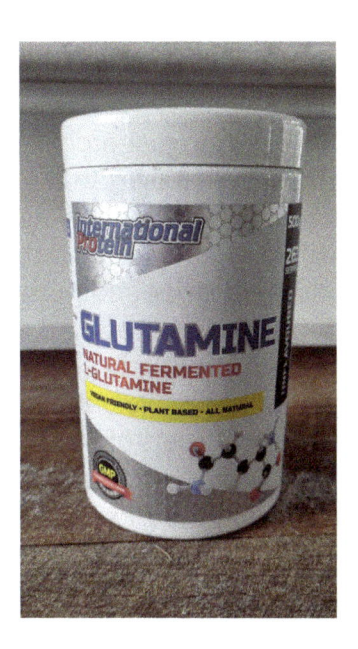

L-Glutamine

L-Glutamine is an amino acid that is primarily used by the body for muscle repair and restoring your gut lining. It also has secondary metabolic and immune functions. Due to its importance, the body can create its own supply of glutamine. However, in times of stress, exertion, or a viral infection, glutamine supplementation is recommended to promote a faster recovery.

Whether you're experiencing severe symptoms or coming back to exercise and intend to get back in the gym, supplementing with L-Glutamine will help take the load off your body's own production of this amino acid. It also produces a relaxing effect on the body by lowering inflammation in the gut lining, which sends a calming signal to the brain that all is well. L- Glutamine is great for consuming in the evening.

For a long period of time in my recovery, I was experiencing pain in the left side of my abdomen whenever I exerted myself physically or mentally. I couldn't figure out what was going on and all the vitamin supplements I was taking weren't improving it. I visited the doctor and explained the symptoms, to which he stated it was likely irritable bowel syndrome brought on by the virus.

With that knowledge, I began researching how to improve my gut lining and what may be causing these symptoms. Several sources suggested trying L-Glutamine as it strengthens the barrier between the inside of the body and the digestive tract. I visited my local supplement store and purchased a large tub of the highest quality L-Glutamine they had and began consuming it straight away with water. Within seconds, I felt relief in my abdomen, like a fire was being extinguished. Excited by the discovery, I made it a regular part of my daily routine, drinking it in the morning and after dinner to soothe me to sleep. I consumed 5g of L-Glutamine in the morning and evening for two months and saw a great improvement in my IBS. I now keep it as part of my supplement repertoire for post-workout recovery or as a relaxant.

Besides being great at calming an inflamed gut, L-Glutamine plays other roles in the body, including:

- A major building block of the protein we need for our muscles
- Boosts the immune system as a fuel source for your immune cells
- Aids in wound and skin healing as it is part of the collagen production process
- Reduces muscle soreness after exercise

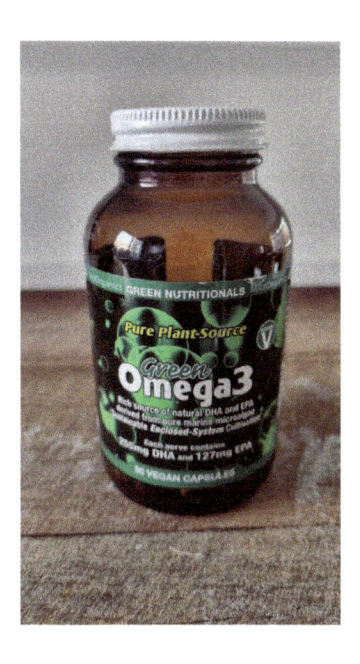

Algae Based Omega 3

Algae based omega-3 is the purest form of the essential fatty acid. Small fish actually get their omega 3s from consuming algae, and larger fish get theirs from consuming the smaller fish. By taking algae-based omega-3, you're really just cutting out the middleman. Fish oil supplements are notoriously low in quality, with many going rancid and sitting on warehouse shelves for years.

I'd always been a big believer in getting omega 3s from my diet. The benefits I've found are clear and improved vision, better cognition, lower inflammation, and high motivation. The problem was, buying high-quality fish isn't always feasible, and whenever I consumed a fish oil supplement, I never really felt any of those benefits.

For a long time, I focused on eating sardines twice a week to fulfill my omega-3 needs. However, if you've eaten sardines before, you know they aren't the most palatable of fish. They have a pungent smell that isn't office or house-friendly and can't be put into many recipes. I noticed the quality of the sardines I could get was dropping too, even if when I bought the most expensive premium brands.

That's when I heard about algae-based omega-3 supplements. I watched a documentary called "Seaspiracy", which shines a light on the global fishing industry's practices. I won't go into the specifics of that documentary here, you can do that yourself, but it recommended algae-based omega-3 supplements as an excellent alternative to consuming fish.

Motivated to try this new type of supplement out, I did some searches online to find a company that offered an algae-based omega-3 product. Quite quickly, I found a local company that sold them. I hopped in my car and drove to a store that had stock. Making the purchase and getting back to my car, I opened the bottle, and took one capsule with water, and waited to feel the effects. Within minutes, I felt sharper in my mind, my niggling lower back injury felt better, and my mood had improved too.

Very happy with the product, and I made it a regular part of my supplement regime. I also found it makes a great addition to a pre-workout stack, lowering inflammation and strengthening blood vessels to maximise blood flow to muscles.

Algae-based Omega-3 helps to offset the high amounts of Omega 6 in our diets. As I stated earlier, we need both in a ratio, but too much Omega 6 causes inflammatory issues. An inflamed vasculature system is the beginning of mitochondrial dysfunction and chronic fatigue syndrome.

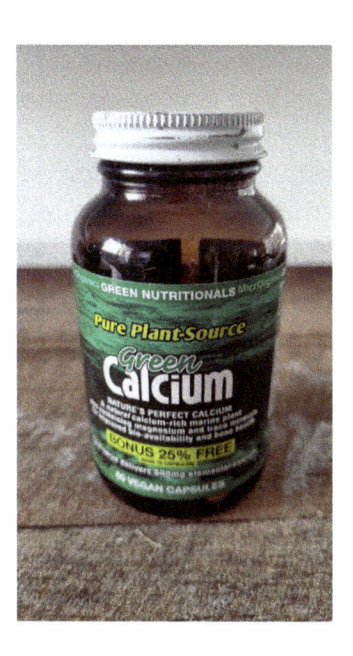

Marine Sourced Calcium

As mentioned earlier, the most absorbable calcium in supplement form is sourced from the sea. Lithothamnium calcareum (search the Internet for marine sourced calcium) is a sea plant naturally rich in calcium, magnesium, iodine, and 72 trace minerals that help with the absorption of calcium.

For a long time, I was winging it with my calcium intake. Eating a bit of cheese here and there, grabbing a handful of almonds every now and then or hoping my leafy greens intake would make up my recommended daily intake. Since I'd lowered my dairy consumption to as low as possible, I was becoming deficient in calcium.

It wasn't until one day, as I was filling out my food diary on Cronometer that I noticed I had barely gotten 50% of my RDI for calcium for an entire week. Curious, I began searching the internet for symptoms of low calcium. Poor tooth health and difficulty sleeping were among the symptoms that stood out to me. For years, I'd been having trouble sleeping; everything I'd tried worked for a bit, but never fixed the problem.

I knew traditional calcium supplements were a scam, as the most common calcium that is used for supplements is calcium carbonate, another poorly absorbed version of the essential mineral. But the marine-sourced calcium stood out as I'd never heard of a calcium source coming from the ocean.

I found a company that listed their products at a local health food store. I bought myself a bottle and downed a capsule just before dinner. Within minutes, I felt my whole body relax and my mood lift. As I sat down after dinner to watch TV, I felt the most at ease I'd felt in a long time. The sleep that night was amazing, no disruptions, and I woke up feeling refreshed.

Besides the highly bioavailable calcium in this product, here is a list of some of its other benefits:

- A great source of bioavailable magnesium
- High levels of iodine to help your thyroid
- Contains prebiotic fibers to feed good gut bacteria
- Trace minerals that work synergistically with calcium for better absorption and bone health

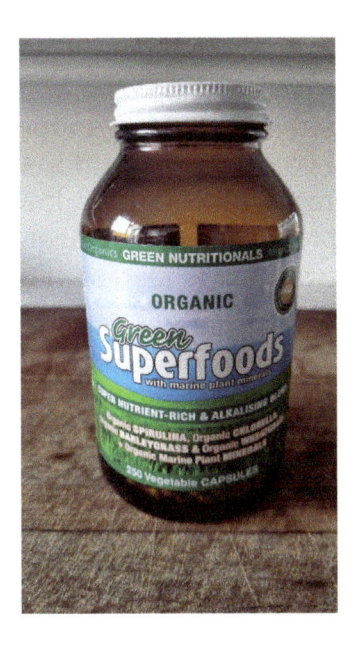

Greens Powders

As I've previously stated, there are several highly nutritious plants that are packed with vitamins, minerals, and phytonutrients. The most popular are spirulina, wheatgrass, barley grass, and chlorella. These are easy to find and can be added to smoothies or just with water on their own. Their high levels of chlorophyll (the stuff that makes them green) cleans the blood and is a great detoxifier.

Early on, when I was battling CFS from EBV, I went through a bad crash where I was bedridden for four days. I was running a high temperature, delirious, and was frankly a little scared. Not wanting to eat anything, my mind was racing to find something that I could take to relieve my symptoms. I somehow made it upstairs to the pantry and found a tub of greens powder I'd bought a few months before I got sick. Desperate to try anything, I quickly scooped up some powder and mixed it with water, swallowing it all down and returning to bed. Within a few minutes, I could feel the chaos inside my body easing, and my symptoms starting to become tolerable. I drifted off to sleep and woke up a few hours later feeling much clearer than before.

Since that day I've included a high-quality greens powder in my routine. Whenever I feel run down or like a cold is coming on, I'll mix up a smoothie with a few spoonfuls of my favourite greens powder and lie on the couch for a few hours. It won't cure an infection immediately, but it will lower the inflammation in your body while providing a substantial amount of nutrients to give your immune system a head start.

While green powders made from these vegetables are a great way to get vitamins, minerals and antioxidants, they shouldn't be considered a silver bullet and not substituted for eating a diet rich in vegetables. Think of them like the star player on a sporting team. Highly effective, but still needs their teammates to win.

When used strategically in conjunction with other solid foods, green powders are a great addition to your arsenal for fighting chronic inflammation and persistent viruses. Below is a list of the major benefits:

- Rich in nearly all vitamins and minerals
- High in protein, especially if it contains spirulina (a complete protein)
- Source of fiber to feed your gut microbes and rebuild your intestinal lining
- High in chlorophyll to detoxify your organs and blood
- Loaded with antioxidants to protect your cells and reduce inflammation

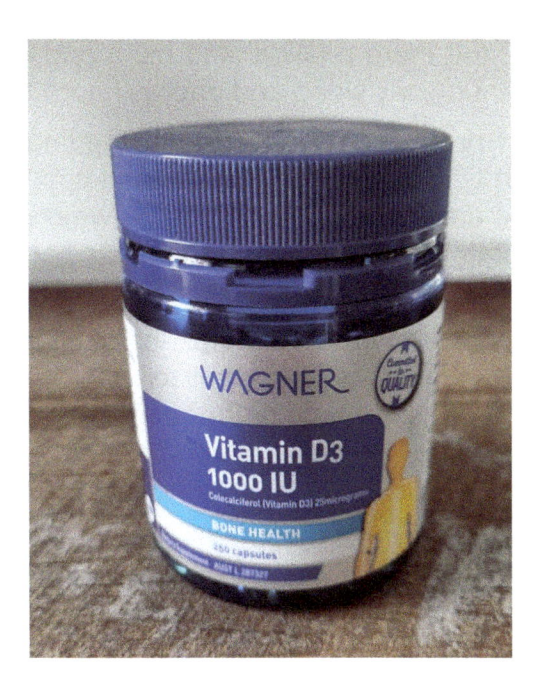

Vitamin D3

If you live in a part of the world that gets little sun exposure, supplementing with vitamin D3 is essential for a healthy body and immune system. The oil-based capsules or sprays are best absorbed by our bodies. The tablets aren't as well absorbed but are a good alternative to not getting any at all.

Vitamin D3 plays many roles in the body. It's especially important for treating Long-Covid because it helps to regulate the immune system. A study found that supplementing vitamin D3 decreased inflammation, reduced cytokines, and stabilized hyperactive mast cells from damaging the body.

When I started working in an office towards the end of university, I noticed I wasn't getting as much sun exposure as I was used to. That spring in Australia was a particularly cloudy one, so even during my lunch breaks when I could go outside, I wasn't getting enough vitamin D.

One night, I was raiding my parent's vitamin drawer and found a bottle of vitamin D tablets. Excited to try them out, I took two with water and waited to see what happened. Almost immediately, I felt more relaxed, and my mood increased. As the weeks went on, my sleep and energy improved, too.

Personally, I prefer going outside and getting a bit of sun for my vitamin D. It feels great and doesn't cost me anything. Though, there are times when it rains for weeks on end, and that's when vitamin D3 supplements come in handy.

Vitamin D3 has a multi-role function in the body. In the cases of fighting chronic viral symptoms, its most important role is activating immune cells to neutralize live virus. However, it also helps to modulate the immune response, preventing excessive "friendly fire" from the immune system and alleviating symptoms.

Some other benefits include:

- Signals calcium to be absorbed from food and be directed to bones and teeth
- Assists with nerve transmission and muscle function, helping with coordinated movement and muscle repair
- Acts like a switch that turns on genes involved with cell growth. It is essential for maintaining healthy cellular function throughout the body
- Sun exposure increases and modulates dopamine and serotonin, two important neurotransmitters that boost mental health
- Sun exposure also regulates your circadian rhythm. Getting sun throughout the day will help you go to bed on time and wake up when you need to

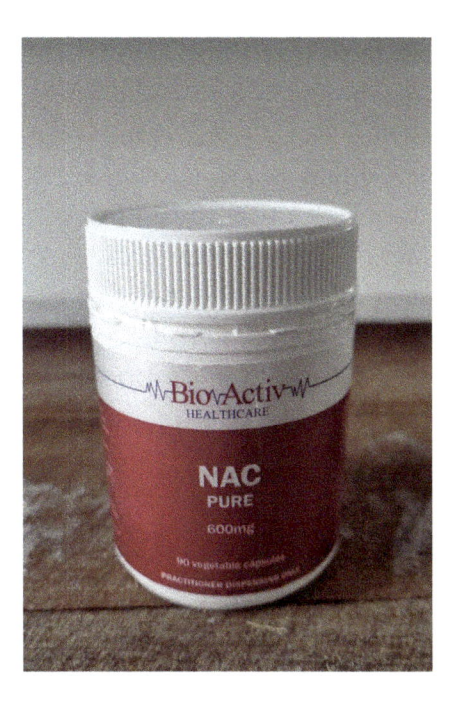

NAC (N-Acetyl Cysteine)

A fairly unknown supplement until Covid arrived, NAC works by ramping up the body's own production of glutathione, a powerful antioxidant. NAC also reduces lung inflammation and mucus build-up. When I was battling long Covid, my lung capacity had been impaired badly. Whenever I breathed in, it felt like my right lung had atrophied by about 50%.

After a few months of little progress recovering, I was faced with another long recovery to get back to exercising and playing sports. Barely being able to walk down my street, I dreaded thinking about how long this recovery would take, as I remembered the years it took to recover from EBV.

One day at work, I mentioned my symptoms to my boss in passing conversation. He recommended NAC as a supplement to improve lung function and to treat long Covid. That night, I went by my local health store and purchased a small tub to try. Almost immediately, the fire in my lungs started to ease, and that lingering sense that my body was fighting a losing battle was over. Feeling a tinge of hope again, I began taking NAC

3 times a day for a few weeks and saw considerable improvements in my energy and stress tolerance.

Within three months, I was back on the basketball court playing with my friends again. I certainly wasn't the same as I was pre-long-Covid, but it felt great to run freely and not feel like I was suffocating.

Since then, I've reduced my dose of NAC to only after a workout or if I am feeling particularly run down. This prevents any flare-ups after exercise and gets my body back on track.

Besides its strong immune system boosting properties, NAC helps with detoxifying your organs. The liver in particular can get bogged down with processing viral particles and other toxins while shedding a virus. NAC helps to eliminate these harmful substances.

It's also been shown to help with brain function by regulating glutamate levels and protecting against oxidative damage. There have been studies suggesting it could be beneficials for conditions like Alzheimer's and Parkinson's disease.

Other benefits of NAC include:
- Regulating blood sugars and insulin sensitivity
- Improving fertility in both men and women
- Reduces LDL cholesterol levels to protect your vasculature from plaquing

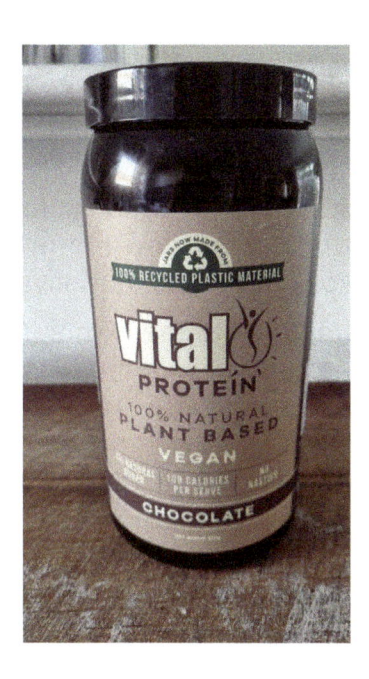

Pea Protein

I was once a heavy consumer of milk-based proteins such as whey and casein. While easy to find and cheap to buy, these proteins are produced from cow milk and can cause issues with the lymphatic system, digestion, and increase inflammation. The only alternative protein powder I've found to be worth changing to is pea protein. It doesn't cause any digestive issues, and when well produced, it tastes great and contains many phytonutrients that reduce inflammation.

In some cases, pea protein doesn't have all the amino acids necessary to make it a complete protein. In those cases, companies will mix with rice or hemp protein to cover these gaps in the amino acid profile. However, I've recently found some that contain all the amino acids, so it is possible to go with pea protein just by itself.

One thing I've noticed is you typically need more of it to build muscle and recover. This is because it's lacking in the amino acid leucine, which is responsible for activating muscle protein synthesis (MPS) in our bodies.

For years I had a serve of whey protein powder with my morning smoothie to start off my day. It was cheap, tasty, and always gave me that little boost I needed. When I got infected with Covid, I found after I'd had my whey protein smoothie, my sinuses would block up, and I'd get brain fog for the rest of the day. Feeling dismayed, I went down to my supplement store and spoke with the owner about alternatives.

I explained my symptoms to the owner of the store, and he assured me that pea protein was the least inflammatory and gave the fewest people digestive issues out of all his protein supplements. He then told me that he was happy for me to try any of his vegan protein powders out and swap them over for something else if I wasn't happy.

With that promise, I went on to try about six different brands of vegan protein powder. First, the common pea and rice blend, but that made me bloated and slow. Then I tried faba bean and rice protein powder, that wasn't much better. Then I found a pea and hemp powder, which I liked, but it made me a little crazy in the head somehow (perhaps that's why I liked it!).

Eventually, I came across a simple pea protein powder which had a complete amino acid profile. Curious, I took it home and sampled a scoop. The texture was a little grainy, but I didn't get bloated or experience any side effects.

If you experience digestive and sinus issues like I was from milk proteins, I'd recommend pea protein. It alkalizes the body and supports the immune system. Due to it being more of a niche product, it's priced higher than whey protein, and you will need more of it to build muscle.

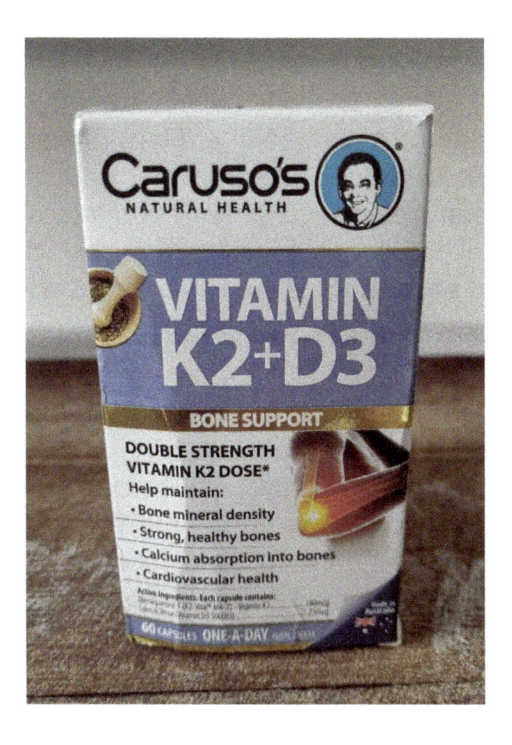

Vitamin K2

Vitamin K2 is a vitamin starting to garner attention from health enthusiasts. Most people have heard about vitamin K, specifically vitamin K1, which is essential for the synthesis of forming clotting factors which prevent excessive bleeding when we cut ourselves. Vitamin K2 has a different function in the body and isn't as easily found in the western diet.

While vitamin K2 has many uses in the body, its primary use is preventing calcium build-up in the wrong places, specifically in your arteries, and moving it to where it's needed most, your bones.

This function is particularly useful for people with arterial plaquing and endothelial dysfunction. In most cases, people with a persistent virus have high levels of inflammation all over their body. Over a long enough period, small lacerations throughout the blood vessels in the cardiovascular system begin to form. The body attempts to heal these lacerations with calcium and fibrin deposits to keep blood flowing around the body.

You could think of it like leaky coolant pipes inside a car. If the pipes begin to deteriorate from poor maintenance or excessive temperatures, they will leak coolant, and the engine will overheat. If the leaks aren't addressed, the engine will eventually shut off, and you'll be in trouble.

In a car, it is possible to tape up the coolant hoses with duct tape or a plastic sealant. But it's never a long-term solution, and the hoses won't ever be as strong as they once were. The human body takes similar measures for fixing leaks inside the blood vessels. It plugs the leaks with calcium and fibrin deposits to stop the problem while the blood vessels heal from the high inflammation. But if the inflammation never subsides, the deposits will continue to build up and begin to cause issues for blood pressure and flow around the body.

This is where vitamin K2 comes in. It activates proteins that bind calcium from soft tissues, such as blood vessels, and transports it to your bones.

Vitamin K2 also serves to protect and heal the intestinal barrier, which is commonly inflamed and damaged from a persistent viral infection. Vitamin K2 has been shown to inhibit the production of inflammatory markers inside the gut and increases the integrity of the intestinal lining.

With these two unique abilities, vitamin K2 is highly useful in repairing atherosclerosis and gut dysbiosis after a severe viral infection.

My CFS and Long Covid never got to the severe stage. Where the inflammation gets so bad, the blood vessels and gut are damaged to the point where basic metabolic functions can no longer work properly. I took vitamin K2 to see if it gave me any health improvements, but since my arteries were fine, I didn't get any benefits.

Vitamin K2 is hard to find in the western diet. There are two different kinds that you want, known as MK-4 and MK-7.

- MK-4 is from animal products, such as grass-fed beef, chicken, and cheese
- MK-7 is from fermented plant products such as natto (a fermented soybean product), sauerkraut, and kimchi. MK-7 breaks down slower than MK-4, so you don't need to regularly consume it to get the benefits.

Like with most nutrients, it's better to get them from natural sources. However, as vitamin K2 can be a difficult vitamin to source from food, supplementation is better than not getting any at all. Always get a vitamin K2 supplement paired with vitamin D3 to ensure calcium is reabsorbed correctly.

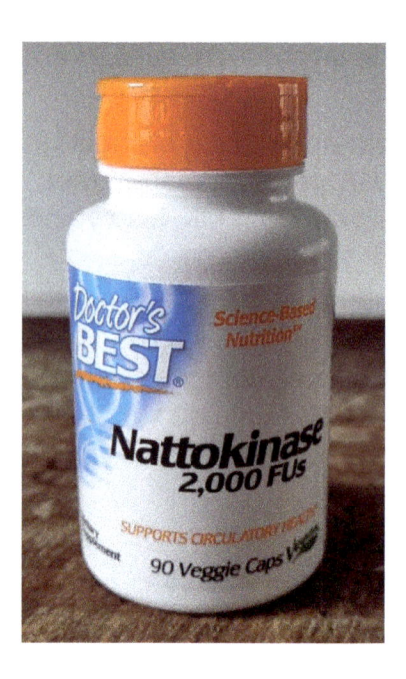

Nattokinase

Nattokinase is an enzyme that comes from Natto, a Japanese soybean and is produced by putting it through a fermentation process. Nattokinase can break down excessive fibrin build-up in our blood. Fibrin is a protein involved in the formation of blood clots, which, in small amounts, are crucial to the healing process. The problem arises when the inflammation in our blood vessels doesn't subside, and blood clots develop throughout the body, preventing oxygen and nutrient delivery to the tissues.

While the body has done the right thing to produce fibrin and clot the blood vessels to protect itself, the modern diet doesn't have the necessary nutrients the body needs to heal from the stop gap measure. This is why vitamin K2 is so helpful for people with long Covid, as it transports the calcium built up in the arteries to the bones where it's needed most. Nattokinase has a similar effect; it breaks down the fibrin that has built on the blood vessel walls and also floating through your blood.

By breaking down the fibrin and reducing the clots, normal blood circulation can be achieved, and the "aged blood" that hasn't been recirculated from the tissues can be cleaned by the kidneys. It effectively helps to restore healthy circulation around the body.

Personally, I haven't used Nattokinase, but I've heard many anecdotal reports that it has helped people with severe long Covid. There have been several studies done on Nattokinase that show how helpful it can be for people with excessive blood clotting.

Studies have also found Nattokinase can help restore gut health. It's still being researched, but Nattokinase appears to have antimicrobial effects, helping to eliminate harmful bacteria. It also is a good source of prebiotic fiber for your good bacteria.

There is also evidence that Nattokinase has an anti-inflammatory effect on the intestines, contributing to a calmer gut environment.

If you think you have arterial plaquing or microclots in your blood, Nattokinase may be an easy starting point for addressing these issues. The low cost and simple administration of this supplement could be an effective treatment for someone with severe symptoms.

Iodine

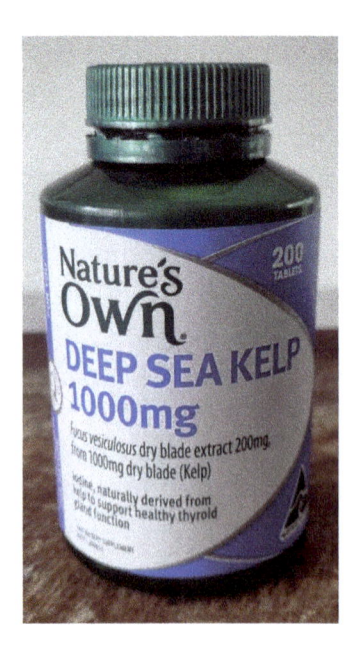

Iodine is a trace mineral, prominently found in sea vegetables and wild-caught fish. It has many functions in the body, including aiding in normal cellular function, the synthesis of reproductive hormones, and most importantly, regulating thyroid hormone production.

Years after my initial infection, when I was starting to get serious about getting better, I suddenly experienced an episode of severe fatigue and weakness. Everything I tried wasn't working. I went to the doctor and told him my symptoms, and he recommended a full blood panel to get some answers.

The biggest clue from that test was that my thyroid hormones, TSH, T3, and T4, were out of whack. I furiously researched everything I could about the thyroid and found that iodine in small but regular amounts is crucial in keeping it functioning normally.

I first tried supplementing with sea kelp tablets. Sea kelp is a large brown seaweed that grows in nutrient-rich coastal waters. It naturally contains high levels of iodine, vitamins, minerals, and antioxidants. Some people buy sea kelp in its natural state and cook it, but you can buy sea kelp tablets that provide the same benefits.

After taking my first sea kelp tablet, the results were almost instantaneous. I got a burst of energy, and my mental clarity was back within a day. I continued to take the sea kelp tablets daily, but after a week, I started having trouble sleeping.

Doing further research, I found that too much Iodine can up-regulate your thyroid function, swinging your metabolic rate in the other direction. I wound back my intake of seaweed products to once every few weeks while still consuming fish twice a week. This seemed to be the sweet spot for my iodine consumption, where I could maintain my energy but not have issues sleeping.

While it's possible to buy iodine supplements, it's much better to get it from food sources. Like any vitamin or mineral, we absorb it much better, and there is less chance of side effects.

Other alternatives for natural iodine are Hawaiian spirulina, wild-caught fish, and oysters. Iodine can also be found in small amounts from land vegetables providing they have been grown in nutrient-rich soil. Commercial agricultural soil typically is void of iodine and many other trace minerals, due to synthetic fertilizer and recycled farmland.

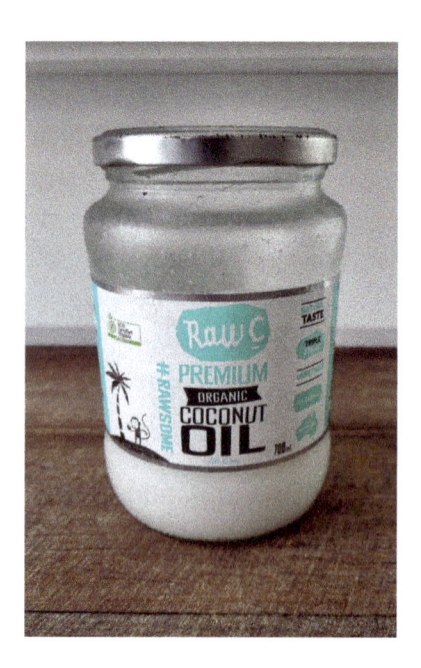

Monolaurin

Monolaurin is a naturally occurring compound found in lauric acid from coconut oil.

It is unique in that it breaks down the outer carbon shell of viruses and bacteria, inhibiting their growth and deactivating them. A study found that monolaurin is effective against a wide range of pathogens, being anti-microbial, anti-fungal, anti-viral, and anti-bacterial. It's also particularly effective for eliminating bad gut bacteria when consumed on an empty stomach.

When I found out about Monolaurin, I went down to the shops immediately and bought the most expensive jar I could find. I began consuming spoonful's straight out of the jar and noticed quite quickly my gut started feeling better.

However, due to my enthusiasm, I consumed too much too quickly, and experienced a crash. It wasn't like crashes I'd had before from over exertion. This one felt cleaner, more like a detox. It was as if my body went through a serious extermination of the bad stuff in my body. Within about an hour, I started feeling better.

I actually found out about coconut oil and its anti-viral properties before I learned that eggs are bad for a viral infection. For many months, I had been cooking my eggs with coconut oil and had noticed I felt better than when I was cooking the eggs with extra virgin olive oil.

Looking back, I believe the coconut oil offset the bad effects of the eggs to some degree. I would say removing eggs altogether gave me the most improvement, though cooking them in coconut oil was noticeably better.

Besides making me feel better and having more energy, it gave me a great focus for getting through my university studies. Everything became clearer, and I had far more willpower for those long, deep study sessions. A study was done in 2015 in a randomized trial that found participants who consumed coconut oil for twelve weeks had significant improvements in their cognitive function. While also lowering their blood sugar levels more than those who did not consume it.

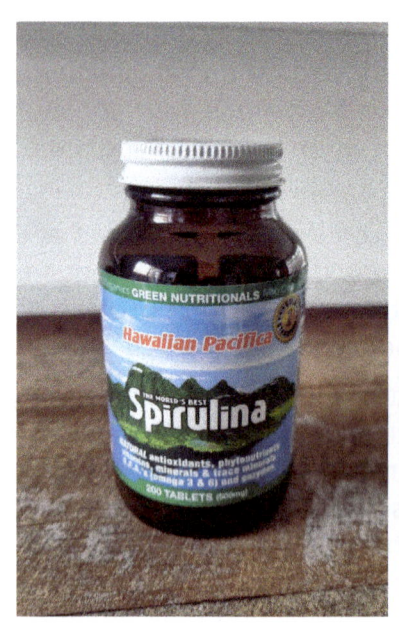

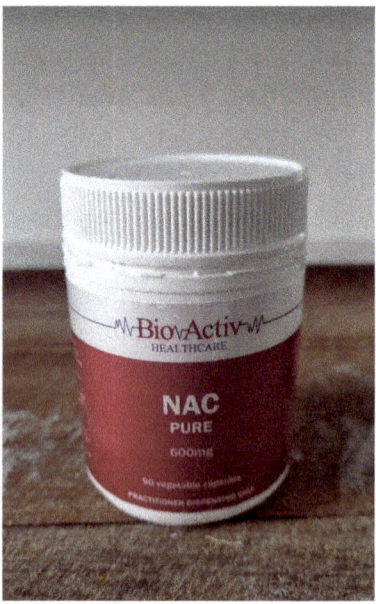

Anti-Crash Combo

The trickiest thing when trying to avoid or recover from a PEM crash is figuring out what your body needs to begin healing while you're dealing with brain fog and fatigue. In most cases, the PEM is triggered by over-exertion or stress, leading to a reactivation of the virus and an excess of ROS inflammation in the cells.

I've found the quickest and most effective way to lower inflammation and deliver nutrients to your cells is combining high quality **Spirulina** and **NAC** together. Both are available in powder or capsule form for convenient administration wherever you are.

Having these two on hand has been instrumental in my recovery. I simply take a few Spirulina tablets and one NAC capsule and I can immediately feel the storm inside my body calming down.

As I navigated through my recovery, there were countless times where I pushed myself too hard and needed a "circuit breaker" type of intervention to stop the PEM. Sometimes, I was on holiday and didn't know where I could get good food. Or I was at work and couldn't take a day off to rest, and I needed something to get me back in the game.

Spirulina can be found in most parts of the world. However, the quality of how it is farmed and processed makes a big difference to its nutritional and antioxidant profile. Consuming spirulina of any kind will provide benefits. However, spirulina grown in *Hawaii* is widely regarded as the highest quality in the world. Here is a quick list of some of its benefits:

- Contains large quantities of every vitamin and mineral
- Has numerous trace minerals such as Iodine and Boron
- One of the rare plant sources of a complete protein
- High levels of antioxidants
- Source of the vitamin K2
- Great essential fatty acid profile with Omega 3 (DHA and ALA), Omega 6, and many others

Combined with NAC, these are a potent weapon in fighting inflammation and invigorating the immune system. While also delivering nutrition all over the body, repairing blood vessels, and detoxifying organs.

You don't even need to be crashing to get the benefits of this combo. Regular supplementation is great for the body and will help raise your recovery ceiling. They also help prime the body for exercise when you start feeling like you can get back into it.

CHAPTER SUMMARY: NUTRITIONAL SUPPLEMENTS

1. Natural Vitamin C
   - Worlds apart from synthetic ascorbic acid. Get it from fruits and vegetables, acerola cherries, camu camu.
   - Heals your skin, vasculature, immune system, adrenals, and many other functions
2. L-Glutamine
   - Integral to healing the intestinal lining of your gut. Boosts the immune system, muscle repair, and calms the nervous system.
3. Algae-based Omega 3
   - Far more potent and cleaner than any fish or krill oil supplements.
   - Lowers inflammation everywhere, boosts brain power, and increases mood
4. Marine Sourced Calcium
   - Night and day difference to 99% of the calcium available in supplement form. Far more absorbable and contains phytonutrients that aid in absorption.
   - Alkalizes the blood, relaxes the body, and is necessary as diary is off the menu while recovering.
5. Greens Powders
   - A powerhouse in detoxification and lowering blood acidity levels

- Loaded with vitamins, minerals, enzymes and phytonutrients
- Try to get the highest quality

6. Vitamin D3
    - Responsible for over 1000 bodily functions, boosts the immune system, and improves male and female reproductive health
    - Sunshine is best (20+ minutes), but oil-based capsules are OK

7. N-Acetyl Cysteine (NAC)
    - Ramps up the production of glutathione inside the body (a master antioxidant)
    - Lowers lung and vasculature inflammation caused by Covid

8. Pea Protein
    - The only alternative to whey proteins
    - Alkalizes the body and contains high levels of phytonutrients

9. Vitamin K2
    - Transports calcium away from blood vessels and into bones
    - Source from grass-fed animals or fermented vegetables

10. Nattokinase
    - Breaks down microclots and fibrin in blood vessels
    - Get it from Natto or in supplement form

11. Iodine
    - Integral to thyroid health and numerous other bodily functions
    - Sea vegetables or animals are a great source

12. Monolaurin
    - Breaks down pathogens & renders them inert
    - Found in coconut oil and coconut products
13. Anti-Crash Combo
    - Spirulina & NAC work great as an emergency crash rescue and vitality booster
    - Highly potent at reducing inflammation and boosting the immune system

CHAPTER 6

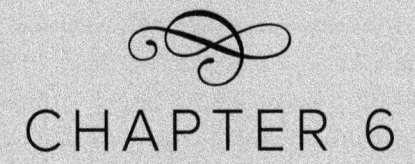

ADVICE & RECOMMENDATIONS FOR PEOPLE WITH MILD TO MODERATE LONG-HAUL SYMPTOMS

The most important lesson you can take from this book about recovering is that your capacity for activity and stress has reduced since the onset of the infection. You'll need to learn your new exertion capacity and be careful not to even come close to exceeding it every day. With time, letting the body rest, giving it the right nutrition, and gradual exercise, you can reclaim your life.

I know most people don't want to be told to slow down. Or they may have a lifestyle that doesn't easily permit this. You could have a house to run or a job to maintain. Someone has to pay the bills, after all, so there can be no choice but to return to work. It's critical to understand that this kind of chronic stress is highly detrimental to your immune system. Having a perfect diet will help you be resilient to stress, but it won't make you invincible.

Chronic stress severely impairs the immune system's ability to recover from a persistent virus. The immune system must hold off the virus while also keeping new infections at bay. Chronic stress can be caused by an excess of work, university assignments/exams, unhealthy relationships, or financial troubles. With enough time, these will eventually overwhelm your body, even with a great diet. All these parts of life stimulate the adrenal glands, making them release cortisol and adrenaline to help you navigate the stress. Everyone has differing tolerances, but we all have a breaking point where it becomes too much, and we need a break.

When you're healthy and everyday life is a breeze, periods of intense stress can be challenging and fun. But when day-to-day life is a slog, and responsibilities are piling up, the ability to cope with intense stress slowly diminishes. It's kind of like a rechargeable battery that never gets properly recharged. The intense demand placed without adequate recuperation lowers the total output capacity of the battery.

I know it's easy to say, "just decrease your stress and make your life easier". It can be another thing entirely to implement. Most people are bound to their jobs, have families to support, or live in situations they can't escape due to financial constraints. What I've found is there is always something you can do to improve things. Whether it's making better food choices, getting that 30-minute walk in after dinner, or removing a roadblock to your recovery, you do have the power to make changes to your life at some level.

While external stress can be minimised by avoiding certain places and activities, there's also the stress we impose on ourselves. Human beings are essentially built for progression and growth in life. When we're not fulfilling this intrinsic need, the little voice inside our head can turn quite negative. Mental health is difficult to manage when we're recovering from persistent viral symptoms, as our previous coping mechanisms may not be feasible anymore.

When I caught glandular fever, I had built up the most momentum I'd ever felt in life. I was studying for a great degree, making serious progress in the gym, and my social life was the best it had ever been. I knew the recovery was generally longer than most common viruses, but after six months of hardly any improvement, my mental health began to deteriorate. I knew all I had to do was get better, and things would improve, but the longer it took, the more my perspective shifted into the negative. My friends and family could see what was happening to me, but all they could do was offer their sympathies. I felt alone, going through something no one else had been through before.

Looking back, I can understand why I felt that way. However, the angst I felt didn't serve my recovery. If you think it might help, I recommend speaking with a licensed counselor or psychologist to help you process your emotions. The mental impairment a persistent virus can do to someone is serious, and emotional intelligence can be hard when you don't know where to turn. I've found it's OK to ask for help from professionals, but expecting support from anyone else is sometimes unrealistic.

This concept is something I've certainly struggled with as a man. I've always believed if I have a problem, it's up to me to figure it out. In terms of physical recovery, there wasn't much help from the medical community, but speaking with a counselor would have helped me with my emotions.

What I had trouble with the most was allowing myself to go "soft" for a period of time. Being OK with not working out, not progressing with my career or dating life. As a young person, these pursuits make up a lot of the perceived status we can attain. It was difficult for me to relinquish my drive to maximize these areas of my life, but the alternative of never getting better scared me far more.

To help with the transition, I had to find new endeavors to keep my mind and body happy. My vanity would like you to think I straight away started learning a new language or educating myself about how the financial world works. The truth is it was a slow process of battling fatigue and letting go of my past life. A large quantity of my energy went into learning how I could get an edge on my recovery. Instead of working out or partying with my friends, I spent my free time scouring the web for whatever insights I could find.

Simple projects were the best way for me to distract myself while I was recovering. As long as you retain control of the progress, you can work on it at your pace without any external stress imposed. Achieving goals and seeing a project through to completion will give you a great sense of satisfaction. Your projects don't have to change the world. They could be as simple as planting a new garden, cleaning your house, or working on a vehicle.

CHAPTER 7

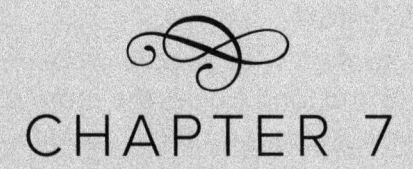

ADVICE & RECOMMENDATIONS FOR PEOPLE WITH SEVERE LONG-HAUL SYMPTOMS

For those with severe long-haul symptoms, everything so far has been about the fundamentals of your recovery. However, in your case, the disease has significantly progressed, and you'll likely need aggressive intervention to get your recovery going. Because the condition affects every part of your body, the fatigue and brain fog you'll be experiencing will make it difficult to take action and change your life. There are medical treatments to get your recovery on the right path, which will be listed in the next chapter.

The more I've spoken with people whose lives have been ruined by ME/CFS and long Covid, the more it baffles me how, even after all these years, an official treatment has not been agreed upon.

I was never completely bedridden, but I was very limited in what I could do for a few years. I can't speak from experience about severe long-haul symptoms, but it breaks my heart every time I hear a new story of someone going through them. For those who are severely affected, recovering with only an optimized diet and supplements will be difficult to break free from the viral persistence and negative inflammatory feedback loops.

The gaslighting you've probably experienced hasn't helped either. In your weakened, hazy state, it's easy to get angry when you hear these things, and your feelings are certainly valid. However, displaying angst and frustration can drive people away and burn up your precious energy. Understand it's very difficult for others to comprehend what's going on with you. Your family or partner are probably your best bet for support. But even they have their own lives to live.

It's up to you to learn as much as you can about your body and try new things to slowly piece together the puzzle. It is possible many people have recovered, but it's not easy.

You may find what works for others may also not work the same for you. That's OK; there are similarities between each of us, but overall, we can be very different. Find what works for you and stick with it.

Twitter/X is a good place to go for information and speaking with others who are going through the same thing. Though, you need to be careful which type of content you engage with as some people will waste your time.

The depth to how a virus can affect the body is still being discovered, but we are slowly piecing the puzzle together. Never stop being curious when you find something new that could help.

For people suffering from severe long Covid/CFS, I recommend a comprehensive approach to your recovery. From my research and speaking with those who had severe long Covid, the course of action below based on the treatments in the following chapter, would be your best bet for turning your recovery around:

1. Apheresis, to clean out your blood of microclots
2. Alpha Lipoic Acid (ALA) IV's or Intravenous Immunoglobulin therapy (IVIG) to lower inflammation all over your body
3. A DNA test to understand your propensity for inflammation
4. Stool/Gut tests to get an idea of the bacteria inside your digestive system and what foods, pro-biotics you need to address any issues
5. Eating organic vegetables (carrots are great for bad bacteria) with lots of vitamin C, glutamine supplementation, and collagen protein to rebuild your gut lining
6. High levels of spirulina or greens powder supplements, NAC, vitamin D3, and K2 supplementation to detoxify your body and repair your vasculature.
7. Getting at least 15 minutes of sun exposure every day
8. If your thyroid hormones are out of whack, then get iodine from natural sources (kelp, seafood) and get high quality beef/chicken/seafood for zinc and selenium
9. Hyperbaric oxygen therapy (HBOT) has helped people reoxygenate themselves and improve their condition. Though, it has been said that if your vasculature is quite damaged, the extra oxygen can overload your pulmonary system.

10. Speak with a doctor about some of the pharmaceuticals listed below.

You will need a holistic strategy for stopping inflammation, repairing the damage done to your body, reversing the negative feedback loops, and supporting your immune system to ensure the virus doesn't reassert itself. The above course of action will put your body on a strong head start for recovery.

If you'd like to consult a doctor that can offer a comprehensive treatment program, I recommend Aviv Clinics. They offer recovery programs where you visit all day for five days a week. They take care of everything you need from the assessment of the disease to a tailored recovery program.

I've also found some cities around the world have long covid clinics. They can help assess your current physical state and offer a treatment plan based on your needs. In most cases, an appointment is affordable.

CHAPTER 8
MEDICAL TREATMENTS

While an official treatment procedure has not been agreed upon, many people suffering from severe long-haul symptoms have reported great improvements from the following treatments. Some people find success in one type of procedure, while others may need a combination to get results.

The issue comes back to how everyone is affected differently by a viral infection. It will be necessary for you and your doctor to look for clues as to what may be happening inside your body and tailor the treatment accordingly.

Some of these treatments are expensive or may not be available where you live. If you don't have the means to do any of these treatments, don't panic; you're not destined to be sick forever. Following all the fundamentals listed previously will help your body get back on track. Though, it may take a little longer depending on the severity of your condition.

Apheresis

The first treatment which I believe anyone with severe long covid should consider is Apheresis. It's a medical procedure that effectively filters out specific components of a person's blood. There have been cases of long Covid sufferers who have undergone several Apheresis treatments to remove micro clots, viral debris, and anything else that's built up from the excessive inflammation and vasculature damage.

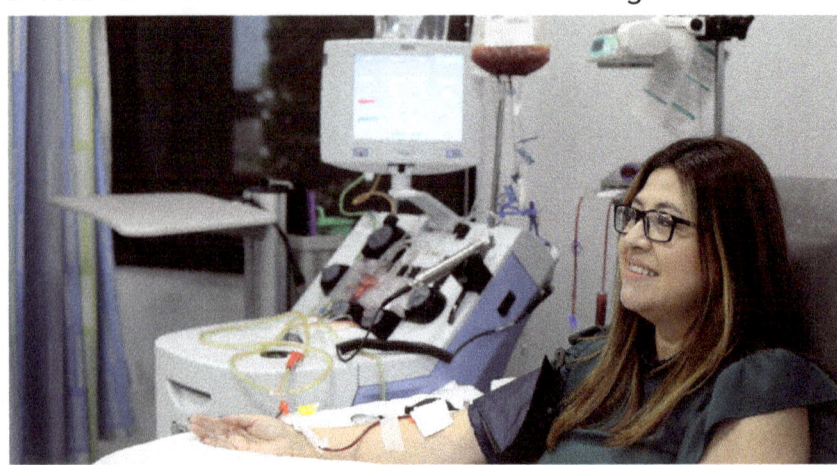

While this treatment may be effective at "cleaning" up someone's blood and is a good starting place, it won't help build your body back up. Ideally, someone suffering from severe long Covid would undertake this procedure while completely modifying their diet to be as alkalizing and supportive for their endothelial health as possible.

The procedure is quite costly, and usually requires several treatments for it to be effective. Most western countries have an Apheresis facility in their major cities. If you live in a regional area, you may need to do some research and look at travelling for this treatment. Speak with your doctor, who can provide you with more information about the therapy.

Genetic and Blood Testing

There are several companies that can test your genetics for various traits in your DNA. The tests can reveal whether you're more likely to have high levels of inflammation, gut dysbiosis, and food allergies.

As you begin to learn more about yourself, you will start to see links between issues. For example, you may be like me, a fairly high-strung person (high baseline adrenaline), so I'm more susceptible to adrenal fatigue. My requirement for healthy food is much higher than the average person.

Getting a full understanding of your body will help piece the puzzle together. A DNA test can highlight what vitamins and minerals you may be predisposed to be lacking and what allergies could affect you.

In my case, my predisposition to high levels of adrenaline and inflammation means I require a diet which supports my adrenal glands and is anti-inflammatory. Have you ever wondered how some people can get away with eating more garbage food than you and still perform? I hate to say it, but some people just got lucky with the genetic lottery.

Instead of feeling envious of these people, which doesn't serve any purpose at all, use this knowledge to motivate you to go the extra mile with your food choices.

A full blood test for all vitamins, minerals, and hormones will allude to deficiencies or hormone imbalances. Think of a full-blood panel like turning the lights on inside a dark room. You can see everything laid out in front of you and know exactly where to go without any guessing.

Gut/Stool Tests

These are effective for people with digestive or nutrient absorption issues. ME/CFS and long Covid can affect the gut because of viral persistence and high inflammation. This can create the perfect environment for bacteria and candida to breed inside your gut, impairing your immune system and disrupting your digestive process. A stool test will allow you to see what kind of bacteria are living inside your gut. You may have a small intestinal bacteria overgrowth (SIBO) issue, or the lining of your gut could have deteriorated so much that you have leaky gut syndrome.

Leaky gut syndrome is where the intestinal lining of your gut has worn down so much that fatty acids and bacteria make their way past the digestive tract and into the bloodstream. These unwanted particles pollute the bloodstream and can even make their way up into the brain, becoming a neurotoxin.

Foods for your Jeans is a company that will take a DNA and stool sample from you to advise the best foods to use based on your gut bacterial and DNA profile. I haven't used this company, but it comes highly recommended for long Covid sufferers who have severely disrupted gut microbiomes.

Monoclonal Antibodies

There have been reports of monoclonal antibody treatments helping people recover much faster than expected. Monoclonal antibodies are laboratory-produced molecules that are designed to mimic the immune system's ability to recognise and attack foreign substances, such as bacteria, viruses, and cancer cells. They are created by isolating and reproducing a single type of immune cell, the B cell that produces a specific antibody in response to a particular antigen.

When I was in the depth of ME/CFS and long Covid, I wasn't aware these treatments were available. The cost of these treatments can vary depending on your condition, the dosage, and the duration of treatment. A full course can cost tens of thousands of dollars and individual doses between AU$2000 - $3000.

Since I have no experience with this type of treatment, I can only offer observations on what I've seen. The people I know who received it recovered quite swiftly without any notable complications. It appears to give the immune system a head start on building antibodies to a virus before it can find ways to evade detection and overwhelm the immune system.

If you can afford the cost, I'd recommend speaking with your doctor about monoclonal antibodies to ensure you don't develop chronic symptoms.

Intravenous Immunoglobulin (IVIG) Therapy

IVIG therapy is like a monoclonal antibody treatment, in that it involves administering a solution of concentrated antibodies. These are sourced from blood plasma donations and administered directly into someone's blood via intravenous infusion.

The primary benefit of IVIG therapy is the significant boost in antibody levels, which are derived from a vast range of healthy individuals and covers a broad range of pathogens. The infused antibodies provide temporary relief to the immune system, kind of like frontline soldiers getting air support on a battlefield.

Another benefit of IVIG is that it has immune modulatory effects as well. These include reducing excessive inflammation caused by a dysfunctional immune response and helping the immune system to create anti-inflammatory cytokines.

Overall, IVIG therapy is like giving your immune system a big boost and reset. Allowing the body a chance to heal and get a head start on rebuilding itself.

I know a guy who underwent IVIG therapy for Guillain-Barre Syndrome (GBS). GBS is a disease where the immune system attacks peripheral nerves and can lead to paralysis. After a stressful house move during winter, he developed a nasty flu infection which took weeks to recover from. Three weeks after the onset, he noticed the right side of his face was beginning to droop a bit, and his hands and feet were numb. Every time he smiled in the mirror, only the left side of his face would react. Terrified of what was happening to him, he quickly visited the hospital, and the doctor diagnosed him with GBS. He was recommended to begin IVIG therapy immediately to prevent the condition from getting worse and to avoid permanent damage to his body.

Luckily, his treatment was successful, and he was back at work within a month. Still, the notion that the common flu virus could spread throughout his body and begin to affect his nerves is unsettling. IVIG therapy saved his life, and world needs greater awareness of this procedure.

I've seen many reports that IVIG therapy is effective at treating long Covid too. With many people saying it's helped them slowly get back to an acceptable activity capacity.

One thing to note is that the therapy is quite expensive. Here in Australia, it is covered by private health insurance and sometimes the public health system if the patient is in desperate need of it.

Alpha Lipoic Acid IV infusion

Alpha Lipoic Acid (ALA) is a naturally occurring antioxidant that is found in foods like spinach, broccoli and potatoes in small amounts. Its function as an antioxidant is unique to others as it is both water and fat-soluble, allowing it to move throughout the body where it is needed most.

Besides its antioxidant capabilities, it also regenerates other antioxidants such as vitamin C, E, and glutathione, making them available for further oxidative stress reduction.

While it's difficult to get substantial amounts of ALA from food, intravenous treatment is available. I have no experience with this personally, but I have spoken with a lady who was recommended it by her doctor. She went on both glutathione and ALA IV to start with and noticed a significant improvement relatively quickly.

In summary, ALA helps the body with the following:
- Helps the immune system restart by dumping great quantities of antioxidants straight into the bloodstream.
- Fight off lactic acid and nerve damage
- Boost the immune system
- Reduce oxidative stress, fibrin accumulation

Due to the obscurity of the treatment, it is likely only the most premium health insurance plans will cover it. Speak with your insurer to see if it's included, and your doctor if it's available nearby.

Blood Lactate Monitor

A portable blood lactate monitor can help you keep track of the lactate levels in your bloodstream. This will give you an indication of the acidity level in your blood and help to correlate which foods and behaviours increase your lactate levels.

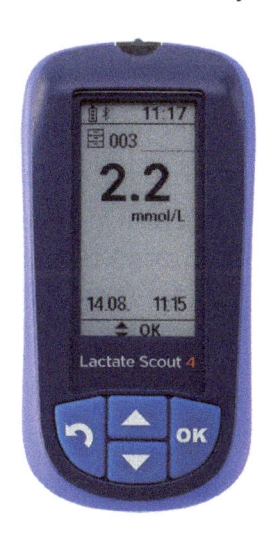

This isn't essential, but it can be a game changer. The same woman who underwent the ALA infusions also ordered a blood lactate test to check for high levels of lactate. The test came back with an unusually high reading, meaning lactate was not being cleared from her body effectively, and she was in a state of blood acidosis.

After her ALA infusions, she began taking regular tests with a handheld blood lactate monitor to get an idea of how she was progressing. Documenting the results of her lactate test every day, she was able to see patterns in her eating habits and activities that increased her lactate levels. This allowed her to identify the foods and activities which were holding her back.

She noticed whenever she was highly stressed, and/or ate processed carbohydrates, her lactate levels were higher, along with diminished energy and lower mental clarity.

Hyperbaric Oxygen Treatment (HBOT)

Hyperbaric oxygen chambers are specially designed to allow a person to breathe oxygen at higher-than-normal atmospheric pressure. This therapy increases the body's absorption of oxygen by 10-15 times the normal rate by changing the pressure inside a sealed room. The patient breathes air like they normally would, and the increased air pressure amplifies the uptake of oxygen to the cells, putting them in a super saturated state.

All the damage to your blood vessels caused by the high inflammation and blood clots has starved your tissues of oxygen. This leads to a state of nutrient deficiency and mitochondrial dysfunction.

Mitochondria play a crucial role in cellular energy production. Poor mitochondrial function is a key reason for the fatigue we experience from ME/CFS and long Covid. Mitochondria produce Adenosine Triphosphate (ATP), which is the primary energy currency of our cells.

If your circulatory system is impaired, your body will have a hard time delivering the oxygen, nutrients, enzymes, and antioxidants your mitochondria need to function properly. As the mitochondria try to do their job and produce ATP, a byproduct of this process called reactive oxygen species (ROS) begins to build up. Without adequate blood flow, excessive ROS can cause oxidative damage to mitochondrial components, speeding up their downward spiral of dysfunction.

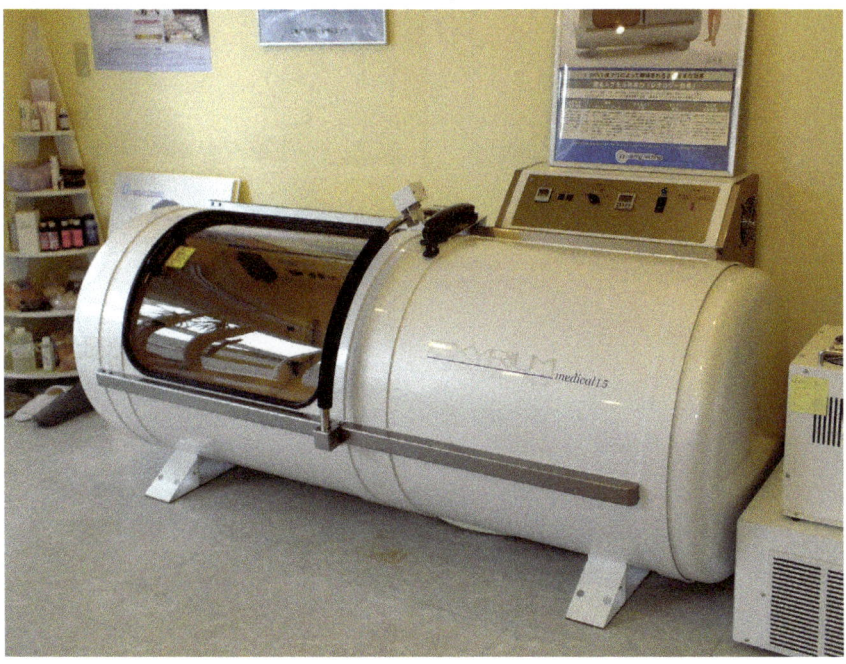

HBOT can accelerate the recovery of your mitochondria and organs by giving your cells an enormous amount of oxygen. This promotes new blood vessel formation, reduces inflammation, and delivers oxygen to parts of the body which have been starved.

It should be noted that people with severe arterial damage need to be careful when considering using a hyperbaric chamber, as the changes in pressure can do further endothelial damage. If you're supporting your body with good, healthy foods that promote vasculature healing, you should be OK to try HBOT, but speak with your doctor.

Personally, I have not tried this myself, but it's a popular treatment among long covid sufferers. It may take quite a few treatments to see improvements; some people need up to 20, but there is no better way to deliver oxygen to damaged cells than HBOT.

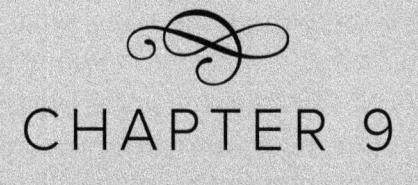

CHAPTER 9
PRESCRIPTION DRUGS

Below, I've summarised the most common prescription drugs used for long Covid; these are either antiviral, anti-inflammatory, or supportive of the mitochondria. The antivirals will target specific processes in the body and shut down viral replication. The anti-inflammatory drugs will downregulate the inflammatory response that may be going haywire inside of you and allow your body to reset itself too.

There are also a series of drugs that work on managing the dysfunction in the autonomic nervous system. Because the virus can disrupt how the body sends nerve signals, specific intervention in these processes can alleviate the symptoms.

I would like to note there are currently several new drugs being trialed for treating long Covid and CFS. As they haven't been widely adopted, I chose not to include them in this book. Speak with me on social media for more information about them.

Paxlovid

Paxlovid is an antiviral medication that works by inhibiting the replication of new viral bodies. There has been evidence that this drug helps in the acute phase of the infection, effectively limiting how far the virus spreads in the body.

To my knowledge, there haven't been trials done on people experiencing long Covid. Though it stands to reason that as the drug limits the replication of the virus, this would help anyone with a persistent infection.

Rapamycin

Rapamycin is an immunosuppressant drug that downregulates growth and metabolism in the body. You're probably thinking, why would I want to suppress my immune system? In the case of severe long Covid, there are many immune system dysfunctions occurring inside the body; using Rapamycin could help with deactivating your immune response temporarily, which in turn lowers inflammation.

In the short term, Rapamycin could help with the run-away cascading inflammation problem. Ideally, you'd want your immune system fully active to neutralize viral pathogens. However, with a dysfunctional immune system, the inflammation caused doesn't always target the right areas.

The immune system is kind of like a fire. When controlled burns of fire are used, it's an effective tool in removing unwanted vegetation and doing back burning to prevent a serious fire event. If an uncontrolled fire is allowed to spread, it destroys everything in its path.

When the immune system is working properly, it does cause a fuss (why you get tired and feel sick), but with time, the body overcomes the infection, and you get better. When it is not working properly, the inflammation increases and spreads to other parts of the body. Rapamycin can help with tempering this unwanted immune response.

Something to be aware of when considering Rapamycin, is that it has a long half-life, approximately 50 hours. It has been reported that it can take up to 12 days for its maximum effect to take hold.

As always, I'd advise speaking with your doctor first to see if Rapamycin may be suitable for you.

Metformin

There have been reports that Metformin reduces the likelihood of developing Long Covid by up to 40%. The drug is commonly used to treat type 2 diabetes by reducing the production of glucose in the liver, increasing the cells sensitivity to insulin, and slowing the absorption of glucose from the intestines.

Metformin has also been shown to have anti-inflammatory properties. It reduces the production of pro-inflammatory molecules and regulates the immune response.

During my recovery, I didn't take any prescription drugs. Mostly because I wasn't aware of anything that was effective. I also didn't get to the point where I couldn't move or was bedridden for days on end. So, I can only speak to what others have tried and share their recommendations. As always, a licensed physician must be consulted before taking any kind of new drug.

Ivabradine

This medication is traditionally used to treat heart conditions such as angina. For some with autonomic nervous system dysfunction, Ivabradin has been used to manage symptoms like increased heart rate when standing up, dizziness, and fatigue. It works by lowering heart rate without lowering blood pressure, particularly useful for those with an excessively high heart rate from minor exertion.

The drug has been found to reduce cardiac workload, have anti-inflammatory effects, and modulate the autonomic nervous system. It may promote parasympathetic dominance, allowing the body to relax and heal.

As always, it's important to consult a medical professional when considering any medication.

Abilify

A brain-modulating drug that regulates neurotransmitters Serotonin and Dopamine. These neurotransmitters play an integral role in the brain and between nerve cells. They are involved in a number of physiological processes and have significant effects on mood, behaviour, and overall well-being.

A common problem with CFS and Long Covid is the impact the condition has on these neurotransmitters. Typically, as a person starts getting healthier, these neurotransmitters start increasing, and you feel better. However, for some, it may be exceedingly difficult to get the ball rolling, and medication may be required to make progress.

It's kind of like a car's motor. Sometimes, there may be so many problems with it that it can't start and keep running. Abilify can help start the reaction and keep it running enough to get you out of trouble.

It all starts with the body suffering inflammation from the infection; then the body gets overwhelmed by the persistent disease. Your serotonin and dopamine diminish, and a depressive cycle sets in. In this lower vibrational state, the immune system weakens, and the body's natural antioxidant production downregulates. Taking Abilify can stimulate these to start back up and help you get back to a positive state of mind.

It is noted that many who reported improvements took a low dose of Abilify, referring to the treatment as Low Dose Abilify (LDA). Speak with a medical professional when considering Abilify as a treatment for CFS and long Covid.

Naltrexone

Naltrexone has been found to reduce inflammation and modulate the immune system. However, it is primarily an opioid antagonist, meaning it blocks the effects of the opioid receptors in the brain. This helps to modulate the pain and stress response in the body. Which is typically disrupted by the disease.

Many people with CFS and long Covid report symptoms of
- Nerve and neurological pain
- High inflammation
- Mitochondrial dysfunction

Low-dose Naltrexone has been shown in studies to release endogenous opioids, lowering pain and inflammation. There also appears to be an increase in neuroplasticity, alleviating brain fog issues and stimulating neuron growth. Studies have also found it supports mitochondrial function as well.

Guanfacine

Guanfacine regulates blood pressure, heart rate, and other autonomic functions and has helped patients with dysautonomia. It's been found to have anti-inflammatory and neuroprotective effects.

A common issue with severe cases of long Covid and CFS is dysautonomia, where their heart rates can vary dramatically, causing blood pressure problems and dizziness to occur.

In a recent study, administering Guanfacine showed significant improvement in all patients suffering from dysautonomia. They also showed improvements in their fatigue and brain fog.

CHAPTER 10

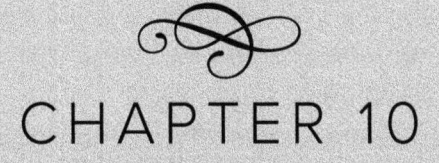

HOW LONG WILL IT TAKE TO GET BETTER?

The answer to this question is highly relative, depending on how bad your condition is. The faster you tackle this head on, the quicker your recovery will be. If you're severely affected, it may take a while to recover, but implementing the concepts in this book will show improvement quickly. If you're moderately affected but going through a stressful time and your nutrition isn't on point, it could take months or even years.

If you only just got infected and scale back your activity while going 100% on the diet, it may only take 1-2 months. Everyone has a different immune system, and we all get exposed to different levels of viral load.

Persistent viruses are sinister. They know how to hide in the body and evade the immune system, while disrupting many critical bodily functions, creating a highly inflammatory environment. The damage done from the inflammation can reach a threshold where the body is incapable of healing itself with conventional practices.

The overwhelming difficulty with these persistent viruses is the uncertainty of how long the recovery will take. It can take quite a while to see any kind of significant improvement in your recovery. It's difficult to know if you are on the right trajectory with your nutrition and lifestyle. It took me years of trial and error to raise my recovery ceiling, slowly learning the principles of health and nutrition that allowed me to find my way out of it. If I could go back to the first week of being sick, I'd implement everything I've talked about in this book. However, understanding my own psychology, if someone was telling me to dramatically change my life, I'd probably only start with a few things that sounded good to me.

This is normal for most people — when you find information that may help you, it's difficult to make the adjustments because change is required. Small incremental changes to one's routine are usually the most effective and sustainable. Anything more, and we feel like our lives are being turned upside down. This happens for four major reasons.

1. Our brains have evolved to be skeptical of people who we have no relationship with. This is reasonable, as you know little about this person, and while what they say may make sense, it takes time and experience to build up trust.
2. You may not be at a point where the pain of staying the same has built up enough to where you are willing to buy into something new that may help you.
3. The notion of change requires a degree of mental energy and self-awareness to admit what you are doing is either not enough or incorrect. It's easier to stay in your comfort zone and not change.
4. Our brains need "proof" that something works before we fully commit to it. It's generally prudent to try something first and see if it works for you.

Looking back at my recovery, I remember many moments where I felt so angry, disheartened, and utterly isolated that I hadn't recovered yet. Slowly watching my physical strength and fitness disappear. I was trapped within my own body.

My lowest point was during a summer holiday years after I first got sick. I'd used all my energy to scrape by in the minimum required subjects for my university course and was lying around at home completely exhausted. My head kept thinking about scenarios of what my future could be like. How would I graduate and find a job? How could I attract a partner? How could I raise kids? What kind of life would I have?

I simply couldn't accept the path I was on. I decided to fully commit to learning as much as I could to recover. It's tough to hear, but if you want your life back, **half-measures will not get you there**. All the small 1% improvements add up, and with enough time, you'll begin to feel like you used to.

There may be people in your life that have had the same virus as you but either had a rough week or two or were completely unaffected by it. I could write an entire book about why everyone is affected differently, but in a nutshell, it comes down to four reasons:

- Genetic differences (some people have a lower propensity for inflammation)
- Their level of stress and health of their immune system at the time of infection
- The quality of their nutrition and lifestyle
- Access to effective treatments

After implementing the advice in this book and getting better, you'll have a far better understanding of health and nutrition than the average person. This will pay enormous dividends later in life when you're faced with new health challenges. If you keep these practices up, you'll potentially save thousands on medical bills and enjoy higher levels of energy and vitality for the rest of your life.

A FINAL NOTE

While I've tried to be as succinct as possible, there is a lot of information in this book. Take your time reading it and come back to it when you find yourself unsure of what to do.

The nature of the long Covid and ME/CFS is complex. The high inflammation causes damage all over the body and requires a multi-faceted strategy to come back to health. Everyone is affected differently, and not every treatment, food, or supplement will work for everyone, though there are many universal rules.

There will be those of you who've experienced far worse symptoms than I ever did, and to you, all I can say is my heart goes out to you. To keep fighting this fight is nothing short of inspirational. I only had moderate long-haul symptoms that lasted years. I can only imagine what some of you out there are going through.

I wrote this book because I didn't have anything like this when I first got sick. Over the years, I've had to piece the puzzle together with trial and error. My objective was to put everything I've learned into one place to allow others to get a head start on their recovery.

How a virus can destroy someone's life without killing them is a cruel fate. You exist to watch life pass you by, incapable of doing anything. Your friends and family worry about you but can't understand what's going on and feel powerless to help. Until governments around the world take this problem seriously and divert funding towards research, we may never see an official treatment.

For those who are bedridden, you will be in the fight of your life to get your energy back. For me, coming back from moderate long-haul symptoms was a brutal struggle, but from my own experience and what I've seen others do, I know it is possible.

It seems as Covid is becoming a routine part of life, more and more people will be put at risk of developing long haul symptoms. As the years go on, repeat infections could restart the whole nightmare for some people and regress their progress.

This is why it'll be important moving forward that we, as a society, increase our knowledge of our health to prevent these outbreaks from continuing to happen. Whether you believe the current vaccines are effective is beside the point; all viruses continue to mutate into new strains, and scientists will always be playing catch up in vaccine efficacy.

If treated early and effectively, the condition is easy to recover from. Even for people with a higher risk of developing the disease.

The most important advice you can take from this book is to lower your stress, stop doing things that promote inflammation, and give your body the nutritional resources it needs to purge itself and heal from the damage done.

You will inevitably experience setbacks as you test new things out while trying to expand your limits. Don't feel discouraged, though; I went through many ups and downs as I navigated my way to health again. We're only human, and managing long-haul symptoms is full-time job. Managing severe long-haul symptoms is more than a job; it's 24/7 365 days a year.

With enough commitment and tenacity, you can slowly start living again. You may have to give up some of the things you love to see progress, but being consistent 90% of the time is enough for measurable progress.

If you have any questions for me or just want to reach out and say hi, please don't hesitate to contact me on Twitter/X below; I love hearing success stories from my readers. If you are struggling with some concepts and need more pointers, then please message me; I'm more than happy to help.

𝕏 https://twitter.com/mikejalcock

Thanks for reading,
Michael Alcock

ACKNOWLEDGEMENTS

The following people were instrumental in my recovery journey. Their work has allowed me to recover and learn about the human body and nutrition. They present medical research in simple and easy to understand terms. If you would like to continue your research, these people helped me the most.

Dr Eric Berg

A master at simplifying medical knowledge and presenting it quickly. Check out his YouTube channel for more information about the immune system, insulin resistance, and keeping up to date with the latest health trends.

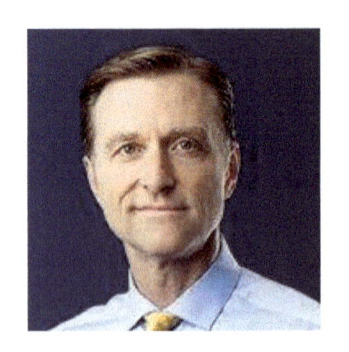

Anthony William

Anthony has a unique approach to helping people. Many of his insights helped me enormously. While he does attract controversy, his knowledge about persistent viruses is unmatched. Check out his "Medical Medium" books.

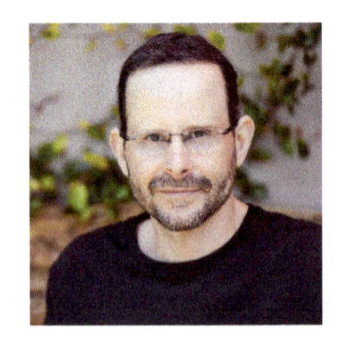

Elizabeth Noble

A Naturopath in Australia who also went through a similar long-haul recovery with Glandular Fever. She was one of the first helpful sources I found when struggling with my recovery, and wrote a comprehensive e-book that started my dive into researching nutrition.

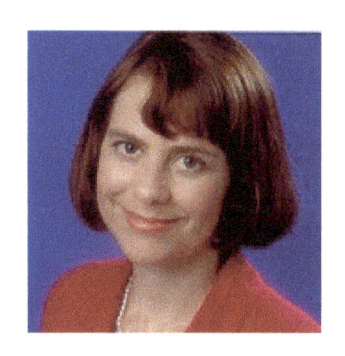

Peggy Schrimer

Expert on Veganism and gut-healing foods, she's been at the forefront of gut-related issues and has provided a range of advice on gut-healing.

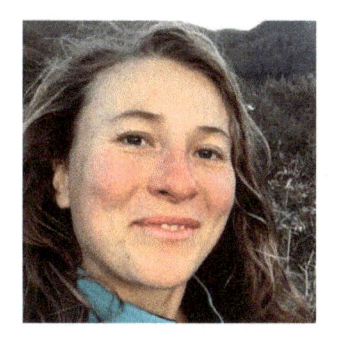

Dr Shawn Baker

Expert on the Carnivore diet, who brought to light the connection between the glucose and vitamin C molecule. Dr Baker is a pioneer in the field of longevity and athletic performance.

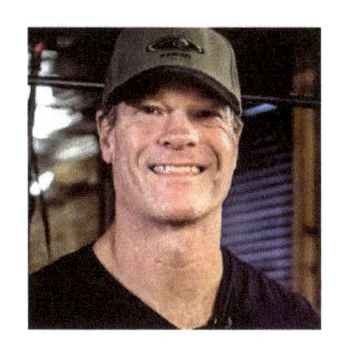

Brandon Gilles

A true inspiration for Long Covid sufferers. Brandon was hit hard with severe Long Covid and experimented with every kind of recovery idea he could find. While putting up a good fight and was showing signs of recovering, Brandon sadly passed away. He will never be forgotten.

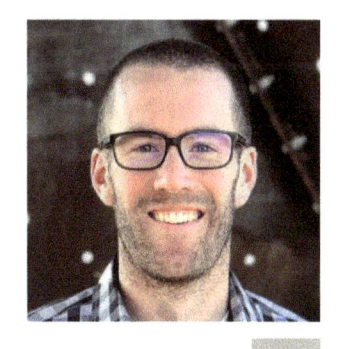

REFERENCES

1. Perlis, R. H., Santillana, M., Ognyanova, K., Safarpour, A., Trujillo, K. L., Simonson, M. D., ... & Lazer, D. (2022). Prevalence and correlates of long COVID symptoms among US adults. *JAMA network open*, 5(10), e2238804-e2238804
2. Zaki, N., & Mohamed, E. A. (2021). The estimations of the COVID-19 incubation period: A scoping reviews of the literature. *Journal of infection and public health*, 14(5), 638-646.
3. Sompayrac, L. (2002). How Pathogenic Viruses Work. United States: Jones and Bartlett Publishers.
4. Medinger, G., Altmann, D. (2022) *The Long Covid Handbook*. Penguin Books.
5. McDermott, M. T. (2019). Adrenal Fatigue. *Management of Patients with Pseudo-Endocrine Disorders: A Case-Based Pocket Guide*, 127-137.
6. Tchounwou, P. B., Yedjou, C. G., Patlolla, A. K., & Sutton, D. J. (2012). Heavy metal toxicity and the environment. *Molecular, clinical and environmental toxicology: volume 3: environmental toxicology*, 133-164.
7. Hu, G. X., Lian, Q. Q., Ge, R. S., Hardy, D. O., & Li, X. K. (2009). Phthalate-induced testicular dysgenesis syndrome: Leydig cell influence. *Trends in Endocrinology & Metabolism*, 20(3), 139-145.
8. Zachar, O. (2020). Formulations for COVID-19 early stage treatment via silver nanoparticles inhalation delivery at home and hospital. *ScienceOpen Preprints*.

9. Williamson, C. S. (2007). Is organic food better for our health? *Nutrition bulletin*, *32*(2), 104-108.
10. Pourahmad, R., Moazzami, B., & Rezaei, N. (2020). Efficacy of plasmapheresis and immunoglobulin replacement therapy (IVIG) on patients with COVID-19. *SN Comprehensive Clinical Medicine*, *2*(9), 1407-1411.
11. Ali, S., Uddin, S. M., Shalim, E., Sayeed, M. A., Anjum, F., Saleem, F., ... & Quraishy, S. (2021). Hyperimmune anti-COVID-19 IVIG (C-IVIG) treatment in severe and critical COVID-19 patients: A phase I/II randomized control trial. *EClinicalMedicine*, *36*, 100926.
12. Yang, C., Zhao, H., Espin, E., Tebbutt, S. (2023) Association of SARS-CoV-2 infection and persistence with long COVID. *The Lancet Respiratory Medicine*.
13. Gold, J. E., Okyay, R. A., Licht, W. E., & Hurley, D. J. (2021). Investigation of long COVID prevalence and its relationship to Epstein-Barr virus reactivation. *Pathogens*, *10*(6), 763.
14. Liu J. (2008). The effects and mechanisms of mitochondrial nutrient alpha-lipoic acid on improving age-associated mitochondrial and cognitive dysfunction: an overview. *Neurochemical research*, *33*(1), 194–203. https://doi.org/10.1007/s11064-007-9403-0
15. Lai, Y., Masatoshi, H., Ma, Y., Guo, Y., & Zhang, B. (2022). Role of Vitamin K in Intestinal Health. *Frontiers in Immunology*, 5491.
16. Sztretye, M., Dienes, B., Gönczi, M., Czirják, T., Csernoch, L., Dux, L., ... & Keller-Pintér, A. (2019). Astaxanthin: A potential mitochondrial-targeted antioxidant treatment in diseases and with aging. *Oxidative Medicine and cellular longevity*, *2019*.
17. Oschman, J. L., Chevalier, G., & Brown, R. (2015). The effects of grounding (earthing) on inflammation, the immune response, wound healing, and prevention and treatment of chronic inflammatory and autoimmune diseases. *Journal of inflammation research*, 83-96.

18. Sanderson, S. K., & Hoppin, J. A. (2012). Pesticides in the food supply: What are the risks? Environmental Health Perspectives, 120(Suppl 1), 155-163. doi:10.1289/ehp.1104287

19. Eddleston, M., Dobson, A. P., & Pretty, J. (2004). Pesticides and human health: A review of the evidence. Environmental Health Perspectives, 112(11), 1563-1572. doi:10.1289/ehp.112-11-1563

20. Sampson, E. J., & Braun, J. (2007). Pesticides in food: Exposure and risk assessment. Annual Review of Public Health, 28, 39-56. doi:10.1146/annurev.publhealth.28.1.39

21. Ibrahim, S., et al. (2021). N-acetylcysteine as an adjuvant therapy for COVID-19. Frontiers in Pharmacology, 12, 736490. doi:10.3389/fphar.2021.736490

22. LaValle, J. L., & Cutler, M. S. (2019). The clinical use of monolaurin as a dietary supplement: A review of the literature. Journal of Chiropractic Medicine, 18(4), 243-252. doi:10.1016/j.jcm.2019.03.003

23. Ober, B. A., Sokal, P. A., & Sokal, K. (2009). Earthing (grounding): Health implications of reconnecting the human body to the Earth's surface electrons. Environmental Health Perspectives, 117(8), 1193-1199

24. Longo, V. D., & Mattson, M. P. (2018). Effects of intermittent fasting on health, aging, and disease. Cell Metabolism, 27(2), 467–486. doi:10.1016/j.cmet.2017.12.008

25. di Filippo, L., et al. (2023). Low Vitamin D Levels Are Associated With Long COVID Syndrome in COVID-19 Survivors. The Journal of Clinical Endocrinology & Metabolism. doi:10.1210/clinem/dgad207

26. Deon, F., Abello, G., Massini, M., Porrini, P., Riso, P., & Guardamagna, O. (2021). Bioavailability and conversion of plant-based sources of omega-3 fatty acids: a scoping review to update supplementation options for vegetarians and vegans. Nutrients, 13(12), 4293. https://doi.org/10.3390/nu13124293

27. Craig WJ, Mangels AR, Rainville AE, editors. Position of the American Dietetic Association: Omega-3 fatty acids. J

Am Diet Assoc. 2009;109(Suppl 1):460-478. doi:10.1016/j.jada.2008.11.013

28. Seth, A., & Singh, P. (2009). Role of glutamine in protection of intestinal epithelial tight junctions. Journal of Clinical Biochemistry and Nutrition, 45(1), 53-62.

29. Johnston, C., & Luo, J. (2011). Bioavailability of natural and synthetic vitamin C in humans. Journal of the American College of Nutrition, 30(6), 534-540.

30. Zimmermann, M. B., Andersson, M., Glickman, M. H., & Braverman, L. E. (2008). Iodine intake and thyroid function: a review of the evidence. Thyroid, 18(10), 1129-1142.

31. Calderón-Larrañaga, A., Martínez-Sánchez, M. J., & Pineda-López, I. (2011). Spirulina and the immune system. Nutrition Reviews, 69(12), 679-688.

32. La Guardia, J., & Barlow, S. (2020). A review of the health effects of drinking tap water and filtered water. Environmental Science & Technology Letters, 7(2), 135-140. doi:10.1021/acs.estlett.9b01033

33. Grandjean P, Landrigan PJ. Fluoride toxicity: critical evaluation of evidence for human developmental neurotoxicity in epidemiological studies, animal experiments, and in vitro analyses. Lancet Neurol. 2014;13(10):950-952. doi:10.1016/S1474-4422(14)70294-0

34. Gardner, CK., Mozaffarian, D. (2019) The Health Risks of Seed Oils. *Nutrition and Metabolism.* 2019, 16 (1), 1-15. Doi:10.1186/s12931-019-0484-y

35. Stanhope, K. L., Schwarz, J. M., Larson, S. S., & Fontaine, K. R. (2016). Sugar-sweetened beverages and cardiometabolic health: A systematic review and meta-analysis of prospective studies. American Journal of Clinical Nutrition, 104(4), 1084-1099.

36. Ahmed, S., Ahsan, M., & Islam, M. S. (2019). Heavy metal contamination in seafood: A review of global research. Marine Pollution Bulletin, 147, 162-176.

37. Joshi, P. S., Kaushik, A., Gode, A., & Mhaskar, K. P. (2020). Antimicrobial properties of lauric acid and monolaurin in virgin coconut oil: A review. Comprehensive Reviews in Food Science and Food Safety, 19(1), 142-155.
38. Agero, A. L., et al. "Effect of virgin coconut oil on cognitive function and blood sugar levels in type 2 diabetes mellitus." Philippine Journal of Science 144.4 (2015): 467-474
39. Francesco L., et al. (2023) "Intravenous Immunoglobulin Treatment for long covid: A Randomized Controlled Trial". *Annals of Internal Medicine.*
40. Barnard, N. D., Scialli, A. R., Glass, J. L., Villareal, D. T., Inkeles, S., Rallis, L. M., ... & Scialli, A. (2013). Fruit intake and insulin sensitivity: A systematic review and meta-analysis of randomized controlled trials. The American Journal of Clinical Nutrition, 97(5), 1103-1112. doi:10.3945/ajcn.112.057594
41. Montefusco, M., et al. (2021). Altered glycometabolic control and insulin resistance in patients with post-acute COVID-19 syndrome. *Diabetes & Metabolism*, 47(4), 1193-1200. doi:10.1016/j.diabet.2021.03.003
42. Brown, G. A., & Miller, J. G. (2021). Mold, mycotoxins, and a dysregulated immune system: A combination of concern? Frontiers in Immunology, 12, 661936. doi:10.3389/fimmu.2021.661936
43. Alcock, J. J., & Connett, P. (1995). Chlorination of drinking water: Health effects and alternatives. Environmental Health Perspectives, 103(8), 683-693. https://doi.org/10.2307/3433847
44. Smith, A., Jones, B., & Brown, C. (2023). Chlorine and fluoride levels in drinking water in first-world countries. Environmental Science & Technology, 55(1), 1-10
45. Grossman, A. 2022. Overview of the Adrenal Glands. *MSD Manual.* Available at https://www.msdmanuals.com/en-jp/home/hormonal-and-metabolic-disorders/adrenal-gland-disorders/overview-of-the-adrenal-glands
46. Lymphatic system. (2023). In Wikipedia. https://en.wikipedia.org/wiki/Lymphatic_system

47. British Fluoridation Society (2012). One in a Million: The facts about water fluoridation. Available online at: http://www.bfsweb.org/onemillion/onemillion2012.html (updated Nov. 2012)
48. Ren C, Zhang P, Yao XY, Li HH, Chen R, Zhang CY, Geng DQ. (2021). The cognitive impairment and risk factors of the older people living in high fluorosis areas: DKK1 need attention. *BMC Public Health* 21:2237. December 9.
49. Green R, Lanphear B, Hornung R, Flora D, Martinez-Mier EA, Neufeld R, Ayotte P, Muckle G, Till C. (2019). Association Between Maternal Fluoride Exposure During Pregnancy and IQ Scores in Offspring in Canada. *JAMA Pediatrics*. Published August 19.
50. Connett, P., & Bryson, C. (2007). The effects of fluoride on health: A review of the evidence. Environmental Health Perspectives, 115(9), 1453-1459. https://doi.org/10.1289/ehp.115-a291
51. De Meirleir, K., De Pauw, K., & Croughs, J. (2021). Off-label use of Aripiprazole shows promise as a treatment for Myalgic Encephalomyelitis/Chronic Fatigue Syndrome (ME/CFS): a retrospective study of 101 patients treated with a low dose of Aripiprazole. Journal of Translational Medicine, 19(1), 217.
52. Wang, J., Sun, Y., Xu, H., & Zhang, Y. (2022). Low-dose naltrexone for the treatment of long COVID-19: A pilot study. Frontiers in Pharmacology, 13, 10.3389/fphar.2022.861589.
53. De Meirleir, K., De Pauw, K., & Croughs, J. (2013). Ivabradine for the treatment of postural orthostatic tachycardia syndrome (POTS) in patients with chronic fatigue syndrome (CFS): A case series. European Journal of Clinical Investigation, 43(12), 1272-1275.
54. Gupta, S., Gupta, V., & Levine, S. M. (2022). Guanfacine for the Treatment of Post-COVID Dysautonomia: A Case Series. Open Medicine, 17(2), e648.

55. López-Huertas, E., Saura-Calzado, F., Vázquez-Agulló, A., García-Viguera, M., Sánchez-Vásquez, L., & Moreno-Fernández, A. L. (2017). Hydroxytyrosol supplementation increases vitamin C levels in vivo. A human volunteer trial. Redox Biology, 11, 384-389. https://pubmed.ncbi.nlm.nih.gov/10736621/